From

Conception

to

Confusion

From Conception to Confusion

A humorous collection of stories from a mom who's trying to keep her sanity intact, her house clean, and her husband and kids from finding her stash of good chocolate

By Julie Davidson

Momosa Publishing

This book is intended as reflections and stories only, not as a medical manual. If you suspect that you or your child have a medical problem, we urge you to seek competent medical help.

Printed in the United States of America

Cover design by Leanne Coppola
Interior design by Susan Eugster

Library of Congress Control Number available upon request.
978–0–9970808–2–7

2 4 6 8 10 9 7 5 3 1 paperback

To my parents,
Tom and Dixie Davidson

Contents

CHAPTER 5

Welcome to the World, Little One 49

CHAPTER 6

Older and Wiser 73

Acknowledgments

Until I met Rallie McAllister, MD, MPH, and Jennifer Bright Reich, this book was just a thought. Actually, a lot of thoughts scattered throughout my mind and on scrap paper and Post-it notes. I thank you both. A million times would never be enough. You have helped me realize a dream. You asked me if I would write a book. And you were serious! I owe this to you. You are angels.

To my parents: Mommy, I so wish I could mother half as well as you did. Your spirit, your words, and your compassion are with me always. What an amazing example you gave me. I only wish you were here so I could tell you that I was listening. I heard you then, and I still hear you now as I attempt to find my way. Daddy, even though you had struggles, I knew you loved me. And that tough love no doubt has yielded my wit and will to survive what life brings my way.

To all five of my brothers: Your favorite sister loves you. And the women you married rock!

To my friends: You have so much dirt on me, so I will just say thank you for your unconditional love and a lifetime of laughs! You are like family to me.

To my birth mother: You made the most selfless decision

a woman could have to make. If you have ever felt any pain or guilt, please let it go. I have had a wonderful life, and I am happy. And for that I thank you.

To my husband, Charles: Did you have any idea it would be this crazy? Thank you for your love. And for your patience. And for encouraging me to write years ago. And for cleaning the basement.

To Miles and Max: I had no idea my heart could hold so much love. You are proof that I am blessed. You are the best gifts ever. This book is my gift to you for all the joy, happiness, love, and laughter you have brought to my life. Please visit me when I get old. Or at least call now and then, okay?

Foreword

by Rallie McAllister, MD, MPH

I remember the first pregnancy book I ever read. It scared the living daylights out of me! Granted, it was nearly a thousand years ago, back in the Dark Ages, and I was young and impressionable. I hadn't yet started medical school, and everything I knew about pregnancy was what my grumpy, frumpy gym teacher had barked out in a high school sex-ed class.

When my husband and I learned we were expecting, we were under the impression that pregnancy was to be a joyous, exciting journey toward building our family. The pregnancy book we chose to help us navigate that journey wasted no time in scaring us straight. Pregnancy is serious business! Women who find themselves in this precarious condition must tiptoe through a minefield of potential mishaps! I ended up reading only the first few sentences of every chapter of the book. *This week, your baby is the size of a plump raisin. This week, your baby's eyelashes are growing.* As soon as I hit the four-dozen-things-that-could-possibly-go wrong-but-almost-never-do parts, I'd simply slam the book shut. And worry!

Now that I've graduated medical school, helped hundreds of patients through their pregnancies, and delivered three amazing babies of my own, I realize that yes, it's important to be educated and aware while you're expecting. But it's just as important to be happy, relaxed, optimistic, and as joyous as possible. When you're pregnant, your thoughts, feelings, and moods have an important impact on your developing baby, similar to the impact of your diet, activities, and environment.

In her new book, *From Conception to Confusion*, Julie Davidson shines a fresh, funny, and delightfully reassuring light on pregnancy and early parenthood. With wisdom, wit, and a touch of irreverence, she helps put it all into a safe, comforting, and gleeful perspective for moms- and dads-to-be. It's impossible to read her hilarious insights and experiences without laughing out loud.

If you're an expecting parent, you need a daily dose of humor. Reading this book will guarantee that you get it!

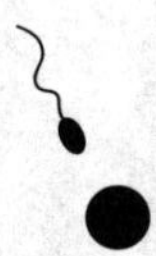

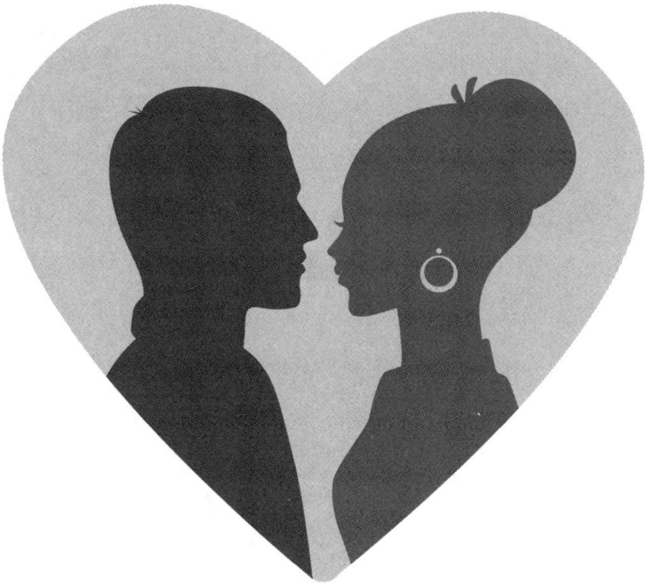

1

The Backstory

THE REASON I WRITE

Please don't be so hard on yourself. As a friend, wife, employee, sister, and daughter. But especially as a mother. Are you doing your best? If so, great. If not, just don't tell anyone.

Chances are at one point you had your life all planned out. Your kids would never eat sugary and over-processed foods. You and your husband would be totally in sync with decisions regarding the kids, finances, and careers. Your co-workers would be happy to fill in for you when your child is sick. You'd have money socked away for all those unforeseen emergencies.

I'm not here to ruin the blissful image of motherhood. That would just be cruel. But I am hoping to convince you that the script (of life) writes itself. We're just actors. I've got a trunk filled with snacks, extra clothing, spare change, baby wipes, and a shovel. The snacks have long gone stale, the clothing is the wrong size, the change isn't enough to really buy anything, the baby wipes have dried out, and I haven't used that shovel in over three years.

Unfortunately for the over-prepared, life never seems to happen in the form, fashion, or manner in which we prepare for it. You will get peed on. Sexy means wearing a shirt that hides your butt. Sleeping in means you've made it to 5 am. Your wardrobe no longer includes thong underwear. It does, however, include a fair stock of laceless, sturdy underwire bras in the gaudiest of colors. Pregnancy makes your boobs big. Breastfeeding will make them sag.

I think we all come into this world with gifts. I don't bake or cook well. My house is obviously lived in, and I can't sew, crochet, or craft a thing. And gardening seems futile; the weeds will just creep back in. But what I can do is string a few words together to tell a story. Hopefully one that speaks to you.

I have but a small amount of dignity left, and I will spare that to share my perspective with you in the hopes that you will see you are not alone. We all have stuff going on. We just don't all talk about it. But I will. I'm the mom who, desperate for pain relief, asked for beer when I got to the hospital ready to deliver my son. I also accidentally dropped him when he was two weeks old. I've taken money from my kids' piggy banks because I had no cash on me. I've used really bad curse words in their presence. The really big ones. I have become so anal retentive that I have scared my husband from the house—more than once.

I hope you laugh. I'd be a fool to tell you to suck it up and don't cry, but in between the tears we need to laugh. Think about how these babies of ours came into the world. They had no teeth, they were oblivious to their own names, they slept 75 percent of the day, and they wore diapers. Do you honestly think we aren't headed back that way at some point? We might as well get some smiles in between now and then.

PARENTING IS YEARS IN THE MAKING

When you were little, did you dream about being a mom? I'll bet a lot of us did. Think about how we started getting ready to be queen nurturers from a young age. All of those dolls we played with. We held them, albeit sometimes dragging them upside down. But we kept them close to us. Constantly.

We changed the dolls' clothing as often as we could. We wrapped them up in blankets. We fed them. Sure, most of their mouths didn't open, but no matter. We tried at least a few times to get some food smushed in between those plastic lips.

We cleaned them. Thanks in part to the feeding fiasco or a Sharpie mishap, we shined those dolls up as best as we could. We washed them with water and dried them off. We even combed their hair. And never mind the fact that many of them didn't have hair. Instead, they had grooves in the plastic designed into fooling us it was hair. Didn't matter. It was hair. Plastic or not.

There were dolls that coo'd. And how cool were you if you got the kind that wet her pants. Score! And some had the eyes that would open and close, which was totally awesome until one eye got stuck. Then it got sort of creepy.

And we had our pick of dolls. Dapper Dan, Holly Hobbie, Cabbage Patch Kids, black dolls, white dolls, Asian dolls, who-knows-what-they-were dolls. So yeah. From an early age, we had that mother thing going on.

And then somewhere along the line, someone temporarily ruined the whole thing by telling us where babies came from. Eeeew! I still have issues with that today. Suddenly, having a baby wasn't at the top of our list. That's okay because attracting boys would replace that need.

So we chased boys. We chased them from elementary school to high school. Then on to college. I still chase my husband, Charles. Actually, he runs from me. Sorry. That's not the same. The point is, we love to love boys. And they love, well: It all comes back to having babies.

I was anxious to talk with my husband about wanting kids when he was younger. At first, he said that mainly it was a quest to get laid in high school. (This is handy to know as we have a son entering high school next year.) Then he back pedaled and said he knew that had always wanted kids, and that vision included having two boys.

WHEN ARE YOU GONNA?

We all have kids at the time that is right for us. Scratch that. We have babies after we get pregnant. Sometimes it's all planned out, and sometimes not. We love them regardless.

It's funny though, how other people always want to

know what's next. You graduate from college, and they want to know when you're gonna get a job. You get a job, and then they want to know when you're gonna get a boyfriend. Then married, then buy a house, then have kids.

I was always sure I wanted kids. Until I wasn't sure. My husband and I were having a good time. My husband says he can't recall what life was like before we had children. I can. We went places. Lots of places. Expensive non-kid-friendly places. We went to Sweden for four days. Partied our childless butts off.

We stayed up late. One, because we could. And two, because we didn't get tired until after midnight. And that was fine, because we could sleep in.

We wore stylish clothing. We purposely bought wardrobes that were cool. Which made sense because we could take leisurely trips to the mall.

We went to fancy restaurants. The type of places that didn't have booster seats or a menu with pb&j, mac 'n cheese, or chicken tenders.

When we traveled, we stayed at places without water slides. Our luggage was just for us and not stuffed with baby food, toys, and a gazillion spare outfits.

We didn't have a budget. We had money. And we spent it as we liked. Mainly on us.

Maybe we lived so carefree because we knew it wouldn't always be that way. At some point, it wouldn't just be the two of us and a dog. I often said that during those pre-baby days, we lived like single people without kids. Just living in the moment. We went to our jobs, ate take out, and watched bad cable TV movies. But in the back of our minds, we knew that it wasn't always going to be like that. Someday, we would have children.

LESS DRAMA, MORE LAUGHTER, PLEASE

Do you laugh much? I mean the kind of real laugh you let out when you were younger. It was that pee-in-your-pants-can't-stop-laughing kind of laugh. The same one that gave you a side ache if you did it long enough.

Watch how often children laugh. They do it at school, in the backyard, at the store. My favorite was in church. How daring, as I was convinced I could get kicked out of church for such behavior. You know it's gotta be funny when you risk being booted out of God's house.

When did it begin to take so much to get a chuckle going? Shamefully, I admit at our home burps and passing gas are especially good to start the giggles. It's a vicious cycle. The more the boys pass gas, the more they laugh, which only makes them want to pass more gas. I know this is awful, but on more than one occasion, my husband and I have told the boys to stop the behavior, but we can't do it with a straight face. We start laughing too. Yes, we know it compromises our authority as parents, but there are times we simply can't help it.

Am I suggesting you go around passing gas and laughing hysterically about it? Not necessarily. But I am suggesting that the grown-up script can be too serious too much of the time. And really the backdrop to our lives—jobs, parenting, marriage, health, and financial issues—doesn't always provide a healthy dose of humor. But how much crying, yelling, and head banging can we do? So the next time you feel that mountain of stress building, let out a good laugh. That kid giggle is in there somewhere. You'll know you found it when you wet your pants or get a side ache.

CHOOSE YOUR ROLE

June Cleaver set the bar pretty high for moms. She kept an amazing home, had dinner on the table on time, and kept little Beaver in line—all while wearing a dress and heels! I'm sure my guys would have thought she was pretty awesome. Sadly, not even teenagers yet, they have acknowledged that other moms are good (aka better than me) for one reason or another. It might be the mom who lets her kids stay up super late. Even on school nights. There's the mom who allows her kids to have TVs in their bedrooms.

And the mom who never raises her voice.

Obviously, you have your own style of parenting. But we can get some cues from different moms.

That annoying, yet infectious laugh coupled with that say-it-like-it-is attitude made Roseanne a household name. Her home was a mess and looked as if it hadn't been dusted ever. And her kids were far from perfect. But her take-it-or-leave-it attitude made her a hero to working class moms everywhere.

Then there was Clair Huxtable. Claire was classy, but she had a little bit of sass. Unlike Roseanne, her house was always in order, and although she was strong minded, she stated her case (as any good lawyer would do) with carefully crafted sentences.

And there's Claire, the mom from the show *Modern Family*. Like so many moms, she's well-meaning, and at the same time a bit scatter brained. She tries to be tough, but when faced with daily struggles of life, she becomes less self-assured.

When it comes to motherhood, there's no perfect equation, which is great for those of us with horrible math skills and poor memory. It's like asking your grandmother what's in her secret recipe and instead of telling you, she smiles and says, "A little bit of this and a little bit of that."

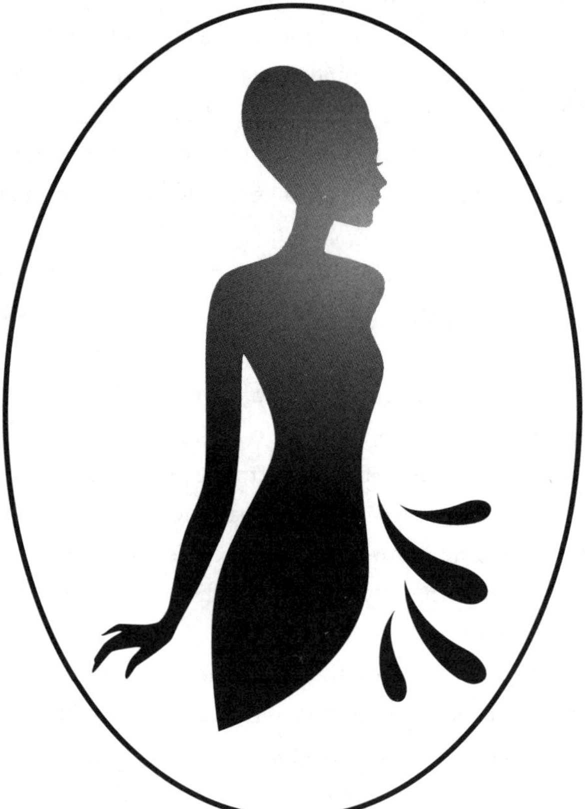

2

Conception

NOW THAT'S GOOD

We were married about three years before we started trying to have kids. Neither one of us can recall when we decided to start trying to have kids, but trying to conceive was a way bigger deal than I thought. Ovulation? Somehow I spaced out on that memo. I had been on birth control since high school. And now like 20 years later, people are yacking away about ovulation. What is it?

Here is what Wikipedia said, "Ovulation is the process in a female's menstrual cycle by which a mature ovarian follicle ruptures and discharges an ovum (also known as an oocyte, female gamete, or casually, an egg). Ovulation also occurs in the estrous cycle of other female mammals, which differs in many fundamental ways from the menstrual cycle. The time immediately surrounding ovulation is referred to as the ovulatory phase or the periovulatory period."

Blah, blah, blah. Yeah. Here's what ovulation meant to me, "Honey. Get up here! It's time to have sex! I'm ovulating!"

Not since my freshman year in college had I had so much sex. Night time. Morning time. Anytime. Now that I was finally "in the know" about ovulation, it was game time. Thanks to my new-found knowledge, my husband was exhausted.

My husband is chiming in and reminding me that I wore him out. It was fun, but he was tired. What I didn't realize until writing this is that he was not excited about sex on a schedule. He felt that sex should be more spontaneous. But, he admits, it was still fun.

One night after a round of planned sex, he turned to me and said, "I know I will regret saying this, but I don't think I can take anymore." Well, 17 years of marriage and two kids later, that problem is solved.

SCORE!

I had the trying-to-conceive thing down to a science. Ovulation. Massive amounts of sex. Wait for period. Repeat until desired results occurred. Easiest formula ever!

Within two months, we got what were looking for. Who knew you could get so excited about peeing on a stick?

I must have looked at that stick a half of dozen times, rereading the directions, wondering, *Is it a blue line we're looking for? Or two blue lines? Wait, maybe no lines is what it is?* This lack of understanding might have been a clue that I was not yet qualified to be a parent. I was really hoping to find a kit that would have a banner that spelled it out. Literally. "You are pregnant" or "Better luck next time."

I called my best friend in a panic and told her I thought I was pregnant but wasn't sure. This is the same friend who and on several occasions has had to parallel park for me, serve as an ATM, designated driver, fashion consultant, and counselor. I knew she would know what to do. Not only did she come over, but she brought another pregnancy test.

Yep. All that foolin' around finally paid off. Until that positive test, practically everything felt mechanical. Like I was just checking things off of a to-do list. Finally, having proof that a being was growing inside of me was the jump-start to an emotional firestorm. I thought to myself, *I'm going to be a mom!*

Charles said his first reaction was realizing that our lives would change dramatically. He began making plans in his mind about what he wanted for our child: friends, schools, everything. And that image we see on television of a father playing catch in the front yard with his son? That image was in the front of his mind.

START SPREADIN' THE NEWS

When it comes to telling people that you are pregnant, there are two camps: tell virtually no one until you make it past the first trimester, or tell everyone, including the bank teller, cashier, and mail carrier as soon as you can. I went with the latter.

I couldn't help it. I was just so excited, and I wanted to share it with people. Lots of people. To this day, I really don't know who I told. I sort of figured that if I did miscarry, I would have to tell people why I was sad and miserable anyway. Then on top of my own pity party, they might make me feel guilty for not letting them in on the big news in the first place.

When you think about it, when you realize that a baby, a real human baby, is growing inside you, you change. And when people around you see you changing, they know something is up.

Here are some of the things pregnant women might do that could give it away that they are expecting.

Rub their bellies: You just want to feel something from the outside as proof there is in fact someone on the inside.

Shop for baby stuff: Cribs, bibs, and adorable outfits are now on a pregnant woman's radar. So brace yourself when you're at Target checking out onesies and you just happen to run into a friend who asks what you're shopping for. You could say, "I'm just looking at onesies, diapers, and cribs to see how expensive they are in case I want to have kids one day." But really, no one prepares *that* well in advance.

Wear oversized clothing: Some people can't wait to get into that maternity wear. Once they know they're pregnant, they start wearing oversized t-shirts and baggy pants, which pretty much says, "Hey, I'm pregnant!"

Avoiding alcohol and caffeine: Certain habits, rituals, and tendencies might come to a stop for some pregnant women. When you order your usual tall, skinny, vanilla latte at Starbucks *decaf*, it's going to raise some suspicions.

Or at the pub if you say, "No alcohol for me, thanks," people will start to wonder. Talking about how you're craving things might also give it away.

Post cryptic status updates on Facebook: This will undoubtedly get your friends to respond to that thread, your wall, and your inbox.

Finding out you're pregnant is one of the biggest life changes you will experience, and how you think you'll react to it might be far from how you actually *will* react to it. Your reactions might surprise you. If you find yourself acting in a bizarre fashion, just blame it on the hormones.

My husband felt that there was an immediacy of getting pregnant. Everyone's circle of friends had one couple that got pregnant first. In my circle, we were not the first. In his, we were. It's not so much a race, but more an excitement about who would have kids first.

NOT SO FAST

Sitting in the ultrasound technician's office, all I remember is hearing the words, "I don't see a heartbeat." In a split second, my mind was swirling and overwhelmed. I kept thinking, *Find the damn heartbeat!* That's what you are trained to do. I didn't do anything with it, so please make it come back!

I just wanted to break down. Have a fit. Freak out. How could this be happening? A miscarriage? I had done everything right. I ate broccoli like it was chocolate. I hate broccoli. I hit the treadmill three times a week. I got rest, stopped putting chemicals on my hair, and didn't go near cigarettes and alcohol. It was such an unsetting feeling.

I sat there deflated. All I could think was, *What did I do wrong, and what do I do now?*

I called Charles to meet me at the doctor's office, and we sat in the lobby with the other patients. We had our heads down, and we were sobbing. At one point, one of the nurses brought us a pamphlet about a support group for other parents who suffered a miscarriage. My husband turned to me and said, "I bet it's a bunch of ladies getting together complaining about their husbands." All I could do was laugh. Laugh and think of how to tell all the people I blabbed about being pregnant to that I miscarried.

Two weeks earlier, a friend of mine miscarried. I knew she understood what I was going through. She invited me over, and we smoked. And drank. And shared our jaded view on life.

The shame and guilt subsided as the days went on. It became easier to go through the baby section at Target. I stopped crying myself to sleep and being envious of anyone else who was pregnant.

I also found out that many people I knew had miscarriages too. But it's not the kind of thing most people feel comfortable discussing. It's too personal, and there is a level of guilt included. Most ladies just aren't comfortable casually mentioning, "We got a new car, and I just had a miscarriage." But dishing on the husbands? Yeah, my husband was onto something there. We don't have such a hard time with that.

In my heart, I knew I had done nothing to cause that miscarriage, but I still felt guilty. Almost 14 years later, I wanted to hear from my husband how he felt.

He told me that he felt bad for me. He said I had this being growing inside me, and he had no idea what that felt like. He was sadder for me and what I felt than for the loss of a life. To him, it was just one of those things that happens. He added that he was shocked that two days later I partied like a rock star at my 15-year class reunion and then broke down after that.

We stumble. We bond. We keep having sex. We keep going.

CHANGE IS A COMIN'

Within a few months, we were pregnant again. For some reason, people like to recall the night "it" happened. It might have been the night I accidentally ordered an apple martini at dinner. (I'm not joking; I thought it was a non-alcoholic apple juice drink.) Or the evening we got a free hotel room. Because let's be honest, hotels just shriek "let's have sex." Especially fancy ones with great beds. Even more so fancy ones with great beds downtown where all the action is.

The point is: It finally happened. Whereas not having a period for almost a year sounds divine, there are so many other things to take its place. There were a ton of things I didn't know about pregnancy. I was completely oblivious to the fact that I would sleep more than a cat for the first trimester. And that my hair would grow at an unbelievable rate. And I was certain that I was sitting on my son's head for the last month of pregnancy. It just felt "wider" down there, you know? Apparently things were shifting. Think about the techtonic plates, only on a slightly smaller scale.

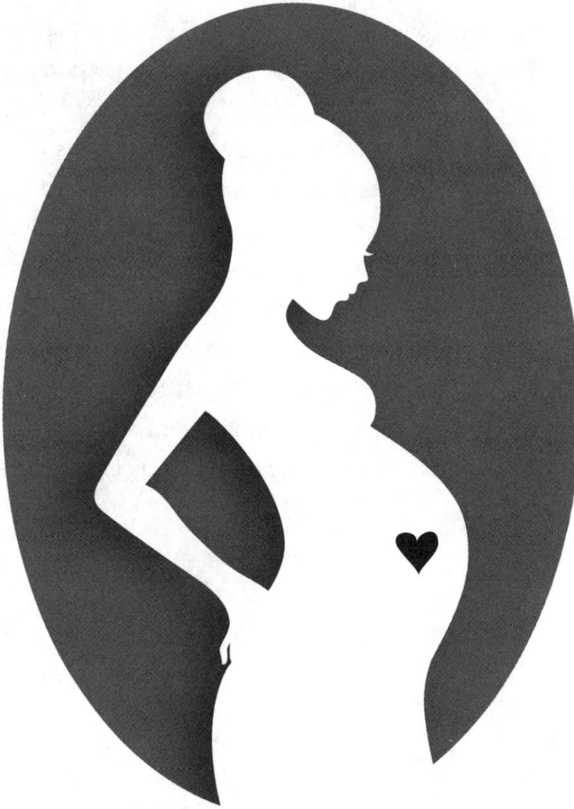

3

Nine Months?

1ST MONTH

Winters are long here in the Midwest. You can spend a lot of time indoors...having sex. Okay, so this is probably not the most appropriate analogy, but sometimes you just have to get back on the horse, and...well...by the end of December we were pregnant again. Missing my period should have been a flag, but something else was a red flag for me. My nipples tingled. That just seemed odd, but it was enough for me to want to investigate further. Not wanting to be unprepared, I had stocked up on in-home pregnancy tests. There are some things you probably don't need to have multiples of, but when you are trying to conceive, you might not really care.

Waiting for that positive sign is very much like waiting for paint to dry. The more you want it, the longer it seems to take. Initially, we read a test too soon and thought it was negative. So I threw it in the trash can. But then I kept second guessing the result and convinced myself we had not waited long enough. I am not too proud to dig through a trash can. You bet I did! I went back 15 minutes later, and ladies and gentleman, we were indeed pregnant! Kinda makes you wanna go through your trash can more often, right?

Month one was fairly boring. It's mainly a time to obsess about all the other months and what's about to happen.

Mainly I worried about the baby being healthy. I wondered if it was going to be a boy or a girl. In my mind, I tried to imagine what he or she would look like. I wondered and waited.

Suspense drives me crazy. I wanted to know what was going to happen and when. I read books. I asked friends. I likely drove my doctor crazy. It was as if I had an adrenaline rush that had me going in a million directions. Nine months is a long time, and I was already impatient.

Do you know how when you buy a car, let's say a Honda Accord, and suddenly you notice every other Honda Accord there is? They're everywhere! You see them in front of your house, on the highway, at the drive thru, and at work. It's kind of the same when you become pregnant. You start noticing all these other women around you who are with child. It's like you suddenly have "pregdar." If there's a pregnant woman within 1,000 feet of you, you'll find her.

The first month of pregnancy is a good time to start snooping around. It's completely new, and talking with some veteran moms might put you at ease. Or scare the mess out of you. There are always a few people around who had really difficult pregnancies. They'll be quick to share stories of constant nausea, weeks of bedrest, and an assortment of ailments. You can take two things away from these friends: First, you see they survived it all, which means you will too. Second, you can avoid them for the next nine months.

2ND MONTH

I have a friend who told me that she and her sisters did nipple twisters to each other. I don't have sisters nor have I had my nipples twisted, but it sounds very painful. Actually that makes me think about one of the first symptoms I had from pregnancy. My nipples felt tingly and sore. And there is something awkward about rubbing your chest for relief at work.

At the end of the second month, I was getting tired. It was a fatigue like no other I had experienced before. It was as if I became part cat, just wanting to lie down 16 hours a day. Yes, even on a windowsill.

Sore boobs and feeling zombie-like. This is when you start wondering when the fun part kicks in. We've all heard about food cravings that pregnant women have. My suggestions to anyone who lives with or works with a woman expecting a baby are 1. Believe her when she wants a certain food and 2. Get that for her—stat! I wanted McDonald's bacon, egg, and cheese biscuits. Not the bagel and not the hot cakes. McDonald's bacon, egg, and cheese biscuit.

3RD MONTH

I think I can. I think I can. Yes, that is the mantra from the book *The Little Train Who Could*. But it might have well been words of inspiration for me to get through the end of that first trimester.

It didn't seem normal to go into work so tired. I was so tempted to call in sick. But I wasn't sick—just half asleep. That is when I realized how amazing some women were to be able keep going to their jobs even with extreme lethargy. I was just trying to figure out how I could prop myself in my chair and take a few short naps without anyone noticing.

Before I got pregnant, I imagined that I would feel great and look cute like so many pregnant women I had seen throughout my life. At this point, I wasn't showing yet, so it all came off as if I was tired and pathetic for no reason for three months straight.

By now, my boobs were no longer sore, but they were growing. If only I could have felt more awake. Sleepy with big boobs. I was slowly slipping into a new mantra: I'm not sure I can. I'm not sure I can.

My husband recalls me worrying. A lot. He remembers me asking for his reassurance that things would be alright. I was insecure as to how I looked as I grew larger. And as I wrote this book, he told me, "I think you looked more beautiful then than at any other time of our marriage." Just wow. I didn't feel beautiful. I felt uncomfortable. But he saw the beauty. If ever there is a time for a father-to-be to be complimentary, around the end of the first trimester is perfect.

4TH MONTH

It was like magic. Once I crossed into the second trimester, I felt like a new person. For starters, I was back in the land of the living.

I remember I didn't exactly have cravings, but my appetite was definitely increasing. And it was quite particular. I never wanted pickles or ice cream. But a few times a week for dinner, it was chili cheese dogs—pretty much the same stuff you had after going to the bars back in the day.

Finally in my fourth month, I was starting to show. Or maybe that was all the bad food I was eating. Somehow when you begin to show, there is a sense of relief. It's like you can prove to the world that you have been sick, moody, and tired for a reason. You aren't just miserable and rapidly gaining weight because it seemed like a good idea.

Pregnancy might very well be the only time you get excited about your midsection getting bigger. About this point, you can slowly incorporate maternity wear into your wardrobe. If you think about it, maternity and children's clothing have something in common. They both might look completely insane on anyone else. But if you're a small child or a big round pregnant woman, you can get away with certain fashions. You know, things with bright colors, ruffles, and bows.

Although Charles had to go on food runs for me, he didn't think much of it. You have to wonder if the guys feel sort of uninvolved with pregnancy because we're the ones carrying the baby. One thing he was taken aback by was my increased libido. Greasy food and sex. Welcome back to college! Why didn't we think of this sooner?

5TH MONTH

Maybe now is when the fun kicks in—literally. It wasn't quite as sophisticated as Morse Code, but it was a sign. There was life on the other side of my belly, and the baby was showing me signs that he or she was active. It felt like gas bubbles moving across my belly, only it tickled and wasn't followed by horrible gas.

You can't help but get excited when the baby moves, and you want to share it with others. When the baby would kick, I would grab whoever's hand was near me and ask, "Do you feel it? There it goes!" Most people were polite and smiled, even though I'm not sure they felt anything.

My husband remembers feeling the baby kick and then becoming instantly more curious about what the baby was going to look like and what his or her personality would be like. And it was this month we would find out if "he or she" was actually a he—or a she.

To find out or not to find out? I truly believe there are few surprises in life. So I went into pregnancy thinking we shouldn't find out ahead of time. That thought lasted all of five months.

My husband told me he knew the baby was going to be a girl. He was so sure that he told the sonographer. Who promptly replied, "It's a good thing you're not a betting man." That's how we found out our first baby was a boy.

Even though I didn't want to find out the sex, once we did, it made it easier for me to focus. Then I knew to stay clear of dresses and all things pink. It was one less thing to obsess over.

However, our obsession with the baby's gender was soon replaced by our obsession with choosing a name. We chose names that we thought were uncommon. We thought we were safe with the name Miles for our oldest son. I cannot tell you how any other boys we have met since with that name. Max is our second son's name. I've realized that 1 out of 10 kids and dogs have the same name. But now our kids answer to their names and have grown into them. There's no changing them now.

Once you choose the baby's name, it's a good idea to keep the name to yourself. Because (like everything else pregnancy related) the peanut gallery likes to chime in. From statements like, "Wow, that's an old person's name" to "Oh, that's different," people find a need to comment on what you decide to name your kid.

6TH MONTH

The heartburn wasn't fun. The only other time I had heartburn that bad was after drinking back-to-back margaritas on our honeymoon. In better news, feeling the baby move more often made me realize this was real.

By now we were really getting ready for the baby to arrive. We ordered furniture just for him. And to think it took me almost 30 years to get a matching bedroom set! I thought back to my parents and how different it was. I think all six of us kids used the same crib as babies—the same crib that would have today's safety experts shrieking. A dresser with an area just for changing diapers? And it took me a minute to understand what a Diaper Genie was. Imagine that. Putting all the soiled diapers in a receptacle that helps keep the stink in! Mark my words: At some point, they'll have that thing spitting out a recycled, fresh diaper for you. This kid had it made.

My husband and I thought that this would be a good time to attend the birthing classes that were offered at the hospital we were going to deliver at. I think the classes are a great idea. But I have to admit I don't remember much. I'll blame it on the forgetfulness they say happens when you get pregnant. But they do cover things about how to know when you are in labor, who to call, what to pack for your stay, and who to call for breastfeeding help.

I enjoyed the social aspect of the classes. You're surrounded by other anxious parents like yourself. You can compare notes and exchange tips.

I recall one guy passing out when we got a tour of the birthing rooms. It was just a room. There was no screaming woman in labor. No doctors. I felt sorry for him, but worse for his wife. He wasn't gonna make it. No way no how.

7TH MONTH

Now I was starting to see the light at the end of the tunnel. It was time to get the whole house ready. I made a list and was checking it several times: Car seat, stroller, wipes, baby gates, swing, diapers, books, and outlet plugs were just the tip of the iceberg.

When you are pregnant, it seems like everyone wants to have a party for you. I had three showers. Not bad for someone who hadn't even arrived yet!

Registering for baby gifts was like entering a whole new universe. There's nothing like waddling through a store with a handheld scanning device making a list of all the things you think your child will need. It was almost more fun than registering for a wedding. Crystal is nice, but this is the stuff you'll use more often.

Before you set foot in a baby supercenter, brace yourself for an over abundance of stuff to choose from. I mean there must be 20 brands of bottles, each with five different bottle shapes and three different nipples. We hadn't even met the little guy. How was I supposed to know his drinking ware preference?

And there were rows upon rows of onesies. Some for girls; others for boys. Onsies with long sleeves. Onsies with short sleeves. They came in solids and with prints. In three-packs or the super duper dozen.

A friend from work suggested that I get a more fashionable diaper bag. I was thinking a diaper bag was a diaper bag. Oh no. These too came in more than a variety of styles: backpacks, messenger bags, oversized shoulder bags, duffle bags. I kept thinking, *This is awesome! I can have a bag full of bottles, wipes, crackers, and teething rings, but I'm still gonna look cool!* Not that looking cool was paramount, but I wanted to be within reach of the "hip" hemisphere.

All I can say is that I hope I have as much choice for my adult diapers as babies have. Rows upon rows. They have them sized for preemies to toddlers. Some have cute little patterns on them in pastel colors. You could make a decision based on price, or you could go with the one that had the cutest kid on the packaging. Or you could be so mired in indecision that you'll be there until security escorts you out.

Baby showers were really fun. Much less stiff than bridal showers. Wouldn't be a shower without games. The one I recall the most was the one with various melted chocolate candy bars placed in baby diapers. Guests had to view and smell the diapers and determine what candy bar was used in each diaper. Those teeny diapers had brown, mushy, lumpy, substances in them. The best smelling poop ever!

Virtually everything that is made for babies is cute. Over and over again, gift after gift, a collective "Awwwwwww" could be heard. I bet no one oohs and ahhhs over adult diapers!

Innumerable trips to stores and three baby showers later, I was on my way. I had most of the things we needed. I also had anxieties. The closer the due date became, the more I worried—about labor, delivery, and how to handle having a newborn.

8TH MONTH

Now I could feel things shifting "down there." My hips were definitely spreading. I felt like an interactive display in the geology portion of a museum. Like when they show what happened to the Earth during pre-historic times. Things move apart—way apart.

I swear that I was sitting on the baby's head during the last two months. I felt like he was right there, ready to come out, and I kept squishing him. Or maybe he was squishing me.

To make matters worse, I constantly felt like I was peeing my pants. Incontinent and pregnant? The cuteness was beginning to wear off. Quickly. I was still very much excited for the baby's arrival, but I wondered how my body would hold up.

I felt as coordinated as a Weeble Wobble or a turtle on its back. I was convinced my front end had stretched beyond maximum capacity. Like when you put air in your tires, you can only fill them to a certain point. I had reached my point. Charles often had to tie my shoes, and I felt my body spreading in virtually all directions. At night I would toss and turn, seeking a comfortable position.

But at least I knew it wouldn't be much longer. It's amazing what you can endure when you have an ETA in sight.

THE HOME STRETCH

By the ninth month, it's obvious to the whole world you're prego. And people—even strangers—feel compelled to reach out and touch your baby bump. It's like you're a waddling freak show, and people just can't get enough. Only you're not getting paid to be center stage. It's all free.

When I got to this point, people felt the need to say things to me. Anything.

Alright maybe I can't have it both ways: You can't both know and not know something. On one hand, I would have liked a little heads-up on challenges related to this becoming-a-mom thing. On the other hand, I haven't always been keen on asking people for information. Maybe because they might tell me what I don't want to hear. But it seems that worst advice is the unsolicited type. You know the kind that people give you without you even giving them the slightest indication that you want their input? At all.

So before we got pregnant, the advice I received was stuff like, "You should go off the pill now because it could take months after that to get pregnant." Or, "Are you even sure you want kids? Cause you might think so now, but if you wait awhile it might change."

Oh man, once that belly begins to show, you're toast. A pregnant woman is like a magnet for people looking to spew all kinds of information her way. A big, round magnet with nowhere to hide.

Here are some of the verbal rants that came my way. For fun I've added responses I thought about giving but had the restraint not to. Please excuse the sarcasm. It's like a second language I became fluent in during pregnancy.

"Oh you're pregnant. Are you gonna find out if it's a boy or a girl?"
"Yes. We know already that it's one or the other."

"Are you sure you're ready for this?"
"No. We are completely unprepared college-educated idiots who waited 36 years to make the biggest mistake of our lives. But thanks for asking."

"Sleep while you still can."
"Go away while you still can."

"Will you breastfeed?"
"That's just creepy. Leave my breasts out of this."

"You look great!"
"Did I look bad before?"

"What are you thinking about for names?"
"Thing One or Thing Two."

"Wow, kids are so expensive!"
"Yes they are. How much money can you give us?"

"Are you going to have a natural delivery or use drugs?"

"Ummm, let's see. The baby's head is the size of a basketball going through a canal the diameter of a tennis ball. What do you think?"

"Have you considered cloth diapers?"

"Yes, they're great for wiping down the car."

On my way to a routine visit with my OB, I somehow had the misfortune of getting on an elevator with a woman who gave me a piece of her mind. She asked me how far along I was. I told her, but I'm not sure she heard or even cared. She did, however, go on to give me a bit of insight into her miserable life.

"Well, just wait 'til after they grow up and become mean, nasty people!"

Who says this to a stranger? A pregnant stranger at that!

As she got off the elevator, all I could think of is that I could expect to see her and those "mean, nasty people" she was referring to someday soon on the *Dr. Phil Show*.

I think the harshest unsolicited conversation came four days after our oldest son was born. He was born via C-section, I was having problems nursing, and I felt like I was gonna burst into tears at any moment.

The baby and I were being released from the hospital.

Charles had gone to get the car, and I was waiting in the lobby. An elderly woman who was standing about 10 feet away started speaking to me.

"How do think I felt with my first baby? He was colicky for the first six months and cried all the time. It was awful."

I didn't even respond. All I could think was, *Where is my husband with the car?*

Today, I ask for more information. I call people and ask for advice. But when I see a pregnant woman, I try really, really hard not to tell her anything that she doesn't need or want to hear. I usually just say, "You look so beautiful." Pregnant or not, you can rarely go wrong with that.

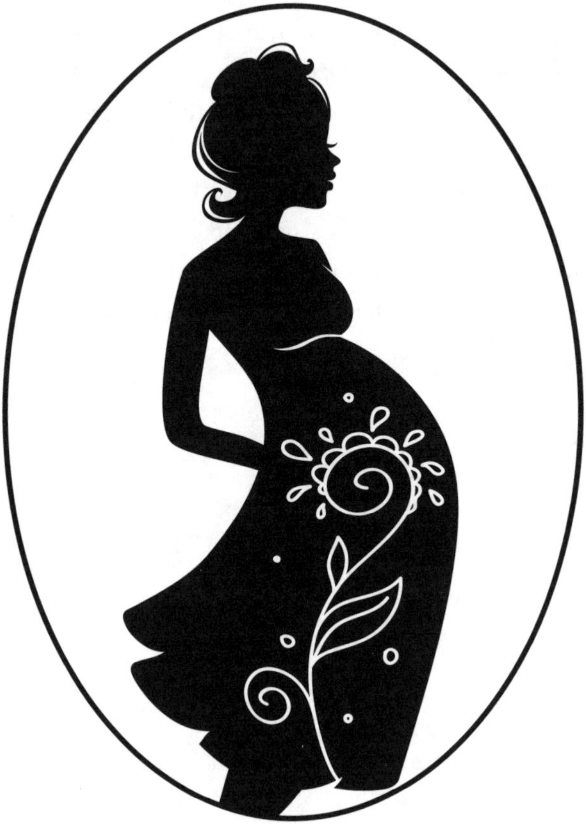

4

Let the Confusion Begin

SHOULD HAVE PAID ATTENTION IN BIRTHING CLASS

For some reason, when I was pregnant with my son I was focused on the mucus plug. What the? It just sounded like something you'd get after a sinus infection. I kept wondering, *Is it like a drain plug? Could the plug get plugged up? Could I mistake it for some other disgusting mushy bodily fluid?*

All I knew was that the pregnancy rumor mill said that once the mucus plug came out, labor was right around the corner. I literally prayed for that damn thing to come out.

It was Friday the 13. Yes. Really. I had gotten my hair done the day before, so I was ready for the baby to come. Because why shouldn't a woman wriggling in pain and tossing around like a fish out of water have a perfectly coiffed do? Never mind the fact that within 15 minutes of labor, sweat will pour out of every orifice of your body, and you'll look like you gave yourself a home perm while running through a rainstorm.

HOW DOES WATER BREAK ANYWAY?

Seems like everyone I knew had their water broke for them so I wasn't certain what to look for. I know now. Look for a pool of liquid to gush out of your crotch area. Then scream. Why? I have no earthly idea, but it seemed logical at the time.

You hear women being mortified that their water would break in different places. Like church. But at least there of all places, people should react in a civilized way. And it would likely be much more entertaining than the sermon. Water breaking at work could be really embarrassing too, but if the timing is right, you could get out of doing those reports you were supposed to do. Or how about at the store? Kind of gives "clean up in aisle four" a whole new meaning.

With the birth of my first son, I think my water "seeped" rather than broke. So I didn't experience that...until son number two. It was 4:30 am and our son Miles had woke up with the sniffles. My husband brought him to our room to comfort him. Comfort was not in the plans. Sleepy, hungry, and not feeling well, he let out a scream. A high pitched, blood curdling, 10-second-long scream. I didn't even have to say a word. It was the look on my face that prompted my husband to take Miles downstairs to eat.

I stayed in bed, tired and longing to go back to sleep. Within 15 minutes, I felt a soft "pop" in my abdomen. I recall thinking it felt like a balloon popped. Only I didn't have a balloon in my abdomen. And then I felt fluid gush out. As that happened, I let out a scream (apparently a theme in our home that day). I called to Charles, "Call my brother now! If he can't get here soon, we're taking Miles to the delivery room with us!" It should be noted that my brother lived almost 20 minutes away. I swear he was there in 10.

THE MOTHER OF ALL CRAMPS

If you have a C-section, you're not missing out on the birthing process. You are missing out on a lot of pain and bizarre body movements.

The contractions began, and it was nothing like I expected. Of course, I knew it would be painful, but it was how it felt that surprised me. It was so intense that it literally felt like I could not breath. I was convinced that something was horribly wrong. There is no way women would endure the pain I was feeling over and over again. Surely, something was not right.

People often say you forget the physical pain of labor. That might be true. But I think what stays with you is your reaction to it. Mine was off the Richter scale.

I hadn't anticipated reacting like a caged animal. At home, I was kicking cabinets. Granted, I wasn't particularly fond of our furniture, but I don't know that it's common to kick fiber board objects in hopes of relieving pain. But at that moment, I really didn't care. The contractions were getting closer, and it was time to head to the hospital.

My brother had arrived and was going to stay with Miles. Ordinarily, I would have had a lengthy conversation about everything from what to feed him to where his diapers were to how to get ahold of us. My thinking was more like, "he can eat whatever he wants, let him roam diaper free, and we'll be back in the next week or so…k bye."

THE BUMPIEST RIDE. EVER

Suddenly a C-section sounded really appealing. I could not even imagine how I was going to get in the minivan let alone endure that ride across town. And there was fresh snow—sparkly, fluffly, slippery snow. As Charles backed out of the garage, the tires on the van began to spin. Not now. We cannot be stuck now. Not tonight. Then a few cusswords from Charles as he rocked the van to get it unstuck. Luckily there were few cars on the road as I think I would have been flagging drivers off the road. I felt every bump on the way there. Every. Single. One. And I was thirsty—so, so thirsty. And there was a bottled water on the dashboard. It rolled from one side of the dash to the other. I was too afraid to reach for it—afraid that any movement would make the pain worse. You might hear advice about concentrating on something other than the pain. Like a beautiful sunrise. I failed to see the beauty. All I saw was pain.

YOU ARE NOW ARRIVING AT YOUR DESTINATION

When we got to the hospital, we pulled up to the ER entrance. Charles went to park the car, and I went looking for relief! Where was the staff? I'm in labor..shouldn't people be carrying me in the doors?

My pride was no where to be found. I slouched over the check-in counter and told the employee I needed help! I asked her for drugs. I told her the pain was unbearable.

She looked at me sweetly and said, "I'm sorry, I'm not a nurse. I can only take your insurance card." I looked around for someone—anyone else who could help. A few feet away was a man mopping the floor. This was not what I had envisioned.

THEY CALL IT LABOR FOR A REASON

I've always been a talker. I talked coming out of major surgery. I can talk in the middle of the night. But when those contractions hit, I was completely unable to speak. Someone once described labor as feeling similar to the stomach flu. I describe it as feeling like a street fight, but instead of fists, hot pokers were being used. That and feeling like trying to do sit-ups every few minutes with your intestines wrapped around your neck. After they were cut down to only six inches long.

At some point, a wheelchair was provided. I couldn't even sit up straight. Sadly, there was nothing my husband could do to help. And he knew it. He sat there with his hand covering his mouth. At one point, I asked him to go in the hall and flag a nurse down. I was in the worst pain of my life, and I needed help. He came back—alone.

My husband told me that the nurses were aware I was having contractions, and they had called my OB and the anesthesiologist. The take-home message for me was that they were coffee clutching it out there at the nurses station while I had fire erupting from my belly.

At the hospital while trying to work with me through the pain, one nurse had to tell me, "We don't scratch people here."

I have never cheated on my husband, but when the anesthesiologist showed up with an epidural, I wanted to kiss him. From there on, it was smooth sailing.

Earlier that day, during my visit with my doctor, she asked when my water broke. All I could think was, *I've been pissing my pants for the past three months, how would I know if my water broke? I certainly didn't break it!*

She went on to say that the baby was breach and was positioned to come out butt first. Now there's a way to greet your mom. The doctor explained it was too risky to reach in and "turn" him. Turn him? Yeah, that sounded like a job for a plumber, and I was pretty sure our insurance wouldn't cover that. Then she told us we would have to do a C-section. After that I kinda checked out. The C-section information was the last part of birthing class, and I blew it off, I guess because I just knew I wouldn't have a C-section.

And there we were. Friday the 13th headed in to surgery. But I practiced my breathing techniques! This was not part of my plan. No pushing while being coached by my doctor and husband? This was not gonna look good on video.

THE BEST-LAID PLANS

Most of what happened in the operating room when my son was born is a blur. Once the drugs kicked in, I couldn't feel anything from the waist down. As much as I thought I was ready for the pushing and screaming, the fast-food-route C-section experience wasn't too bad. Just sit back and let them cut you open.

My OB has the best bedside manner I have ever been witness to. She's calm and soft- spoken. This is quite different from me, who is nervous and loud. She even asked if I wanted music during the procedure.

I thought, *No, I just want my baby.*

Having a C-section was a control freak's worst nightmare. I was bound to a table, physically numb for half my body, and emotionally not sure I was ready to handle what was about to take place.

After a flurry of activity between the doctors and nurses, I heard a collective hush come over the room.

The doctor told me, "He's so handsome. He reminds me of my guys when they were little. If you don't want him, I'll take him home!"

I thought, *Well let me see him first, and I'll let you know.*

My husband was crying and had this sound to his voice I have never heard before or since. It was like a cross between a boy in puberty's cracking voice and a whisper. "He's perfect."

Well, that was all good and well, but I just wanted to see the baby! Someone, please show me the baby!

As I lay on the operating table flat on my back, almost magically the baby appeared in front of me. It was kind of like those flying stunts they do on stage at award shows and concerts. You know where someone looks as if they're floating through the air. You know there's a string attached, but you just can't see it. I didn't see a string attached. As a matter of fact, I don't even recall seeing a hand holding him over me. All I saw was my baby—with beautiful color and smooth soft hair. He was round and squishy. He was perfect. And then he cried. Oh. My. God.

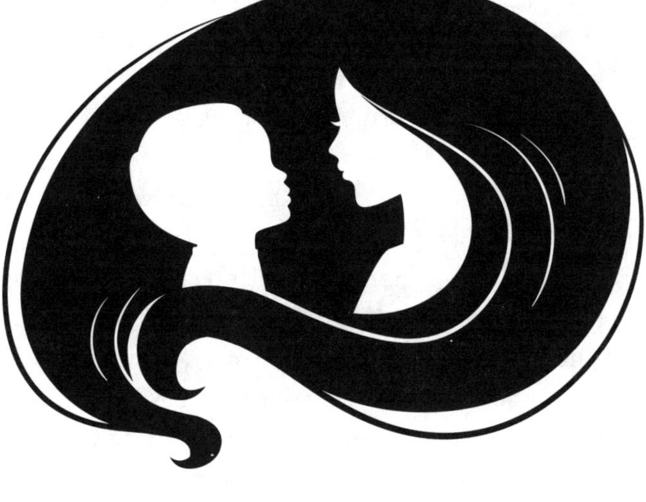

5

Welcome to the World, Little One

READY, SET, GO!

It felt like I was going from zero to 60 in a split second. When the baby arrives, it all seems so surreal. And daunting. And overwhelming. I was overjoyed and a nervous wreck at the same time.

Thank goodness for the help of good staff at the hospital. They fed me, brought the baby to me, got me walking, and tried to assist with breastfeeding. It was my neonatal entourage.

I had heard a ton of stuff about how a woman's body and emotional state could be post partum. But actually experiencing it all is totally different.

When I held my baby in my arms, I was moved to happy tears. I'm adopted, and I was overjoyed to finally see someone who looked like me! As my baby slept, I studied every inch of his body, getting to know everything from his scent to his birthmarks. He wasn't just a round ball in my tummy. He was a full-fledged baby finally in the outside world.

I was a bit weepy and emotional. Although I had a seemingly perfect child, I had this bizarre empty feeling. When Miles cried, it made me nervous. I could hear him wailing down the hall as the nurses brought him to me for feeding. Even though I had babysat and had nieces and nephews, I kept thinking, How long is he going to keep this up?

Each day, I felt stronger. I was getting around on my

own, eating well, and feeling more comfortable holding the baby. And then it was time for us to go home. That thought almost paralyzed me. I really, really didn't want to go home. And not only was it time for me to go home, but I had to take the baby with me. If they could have thrown in a few nurses, the adjustable bed, and room service, I would have taken it much better.

NOW WHAT?

On the ride home from the hospital, I felt a very heightened sense of anxiousness. It seemed as if all the drivers around us were idiots. Why were they driving so fast? If I could have, I would have gotten out of the car in the midst of the traffic and motioned people to slow down. I wished I had a way to let people know that we had a teeny tiny baby in the car, and they need to slow down. I rode in the backseat, one hand over the infant carrier, the other one making rude hand gestures to impatient drivers. Wow, that momma bear instinct kicks in pretty fast.

After our stressful drive home, my husband pulled our car into the garage. When the garage door closed behind us, I felt a brief moment of relief. The bustle of the traffic was over. And then I started to cry. Right there in the garage. That was one of the first moments I felt truly petrified to be a mother. I just didn't know how I was going to do this. It wasn't any one thing in particular. It was all of it. I knew in my heart that I couldn't screw this up, but for those few moments I couldn't find the strength to deal with it.

Once we got inside, I began to settle down a bit. Miles was asleep, so I figured it would be a good time to lay him down in his crib. Everything in his room was in place: baby monitor, wipes, clothes, books, diapers, and Diaper Genie. I sat down in my new recliner. I just sat there staring at this fresh little being. The quiet was almost too much to take, and I wondered, *Now what? Do I stay here and watch him? Do I lie down and nap? Should I wake him up?*

It's ironic how you can earn money, experience traveling the world, and have a great education, but you still have no idea what to do with something that weighs less than nine pounds.

PHONE A FRIEND

There was some freaking out on my part. Breastfeeding was not going well, and it was quite painful. And that parlayed into worrying that my baby wasn't gaining weight. Which made for a tense atmosphere at home.

I had decided that I was going to breastfeed that child no matter what it took. When we were kids, we used to catch baby birds—until someone told us that if you touch them, the momma bird will desert them. I worried about a similar situation with my insistence to breastfeed. I heard that if you started breastfeeding, you couldn't switch to formula. Yep, the kid would be a milk snob at an early age.

The problem was I couldn't get my baby to latch on correctly. It was very painful for me, and he wasn't gaining enough weight. Charles's plan was basically to feed the baby any way that we could. But I was stubborn, and I wanted to hold out hope that I could get him to nurse the right way.

So we did what any couple in crisis would do: We got our relatives involved. Charles's brother is a pediatrician, and my sister-in-law is an ob-gyn nurse practitioner and lactation consultant. After several frantic calls a few days later, all was good.

My new motto is: Be prepared to be unprepared. You won't be disappointed.

BABY HOG

So if you are a woman, you carried the baby. You got to wear cute maternity clothes. You registered for baby gifts. You had the baby showers. You gave birth. You get to breastfeed the baby. You get to take maternity leave.

You! You! You!

But consider that because you carried the baby, gave birth, and are the one to breastfeed, you'll be worn out.

I've heard it said that when a baby cries, something happens to a mom. There's likely some Latin medical term for it. I say that we get weird. The baby cries, and we jump up. Gotta feed, gotta hold, gotta soothe. Then we complain about how much we do and how hard it all is. The problem with that is your husband or partner doesn't get to be part of things. And well, he was there for the getting pregnant part, so it's only fair he gets to be there now.

Maybe you think that Dad won't do things the way you want. And you're probably right. My husband rocked our oldest son to sleep in his arms in front of the television. I kept thinking that was too much exposure to TV at such a young age. My older son is now 14 years old and, what do you know? He's not glued to the television.

Besides, if you don't divvy up the work, then the baby won't get to know Dad and will only want you. From an ego standpoint, how cool is that? Yeah, you are the number one go-to person. Mom is queen. But Mom might want to go to the grocery store alone! Or meet her girlfriends for dinner or a spa day.

My husband reminded me about a time when he could not get our son Miles to take a bottle from him. The kid only wanted milk directly from me. I was working evenings and would leave pumped milk for the baby. Miles refused to take the bottle, plus he screamed so loudly and constantly that my husband convinced himself that our son disliked him. That broke my heart. Fourteen years later, my husband can see that nothing is further from the truth—unless he doesn't buy them cool video games now and then.

Seems like Moms always get the glory when it comes to raising kids. Let Dad help. It's good for him and for the baby. Your child will still love you. And on the days it's questionable, buy him a cool video game.

COMMENTS FROM THE PEANUT GALLERY

Having a new baby is exciting. But the fact is, it's all new. You're trying to figure out how this works. There's no manual specific to your baby. You just have to figure it all out. And rest assured, plenty of people will be around to put in their two cents.

Breastfeeding, daycare, and cold remedies are all up for debate. And everyone seems to know what's best.

I recall an older relative talking about putting a little alcohol in the baby's bottle. Umm, does that seem a bit unhealthy, illegal, and just plain wrong? Now a glass of wine for the parents, I get. I don't remember my parents letting me have alcohol at age 10, 16, or even 20. So why would I dare give alcohol to an infant? Couldn't that lead to other problems? Say, like a drunk baby?

Then someone chimed in about how to put a few more pounds on a baby and shared the advice of putting oatmeal in the baby's bottle along with the milk. This might very well be the reason that I'm turned off by the sight of oatmeal. Unless it's in cookies.

Some people told me not to cut my baby's hair until he was a year old. There are different reasons people give this advice, including the baby's speech will be impaired or he won't crawl. I cut my son's hair before he was a year old. It was a necessity, because I didn't think the sheep dog look was cool. Not sure of what to do with all that freshly cut hair, I placed it in a Ziploc bag. Now, once a year my son takes take the bag out and runs around the house boasting, "This was my hair when I was a baby!" His speech and motor skills were not destroyed by that haircut. Plus, he has a bag of hair to play with once a year.

"Get professional photos taken of the kids every year," was another suggestion given to me. Admittedly, it's very cool to line the pictures up and see the changes from year to year. But that generally requires a cute little dress or nice slacks and a tie that realistically, they'll wear just for that photo. And yes, it is possible that they will poop, upchuck, or destroy that outfit the day of the photo shoot. And no matter how good the photographer is and how hard she tries, there's a strong likelihood that the kid won't smile. All that for around $150. Now we set it up at home. My standards are not high: Wear what you want, and try to look in the direction of the camera. It certainly gives the photos a more "real" look.

When you're having trouble getting the baby to settle down for the night, tons of people will try to convince you to let your baby cry himself to sleep. That's so much easier said than done. When you go from no kids and quiet nights to a baby screaming at excessive decibels, you get a bit freaked out. Those tiny creatures can cry for long periods of time. It's like a recorded loop of the same cry. Only it's not recorded. It's live. In your house.

Best advice? Do what works for you. Even if that means that you run in to pick up your long-haired baby every time he cries.

WOULD YOU LIKE PAPER OR CLOTH?

You probably went in to the whole having-a-baby thing with a good idea of how you were going to raise your child. Ideas are good, but they might change.

Naturally, Charles and I had lots of ideas. We thought we'd like to try cloth diapers. But when I realized someone would have to *wash* all of those diapers, I quickly changed my mind. I just can't fall for the "Oh, it's not bad when it's your own child's poop." Sorry. Poop is smelly and messy. Even your own kids'. IT SMELLS LIKE POOP! If that weren't a big enough turn off, my mind went to how my mother freely admitted she stuck us with pins attempting to get those cloth diapers on. I wasn't sure we could substitute the pins with duct tape. And honestly, I am the world's worst gift wrapper. I couldn't help but think how the cloth diapers would look like—a wad of material on the baby's bottom. Just couldn't do it.

We bought the least expensive disposable diapers. I mean, if they were reusable, we would have spent more money on them, but it's one and done! I just couldn't be convinced that one brand was so much better than another. When the kid fills that diaper, it's gonna sag. No diaper can hide what is inside that diaper. That, my friends, would be a miracle and worth millions. I did find out that you can put disposable diapers in the washing machine. They triple in size and look a bit tattered BUT they come out clean.

My sister-in-law told me about a time they were traveling and their son had diarrhea. They ran out of diapers. They used trash bags! That story stuck with me, and so I stuck diapers in virtually every place I could think of…the diaper bag in the mini van…the diaper bag in the house… my purse….the emergency kit in the car.

It never ceased to amaze me how much poop someone so small could produce. Talk about being regular. And it all originates from the same place but ends up anywhere!

THAT'S WHAT THEY'RE FOR!

We also decided to breastfeed. Finally I could use the girls for what they were created for. I figured it would be simple. The baby would be hungry, and I would feed him from my milk stash. Two steps. Easy.

So add breastfeeding to the list of things I thought I could easily handle. My son was latching on the wrong way. And latching hard. Within 30 minutes of my first attempt, I had a pain shooting down my neck from my ear to my collarbone. It wasn't working, and I felt like a failure.

Relief came seven days after our son was born. My sister-in-law came to help. She's an ob-gyn nurse practitioner. And a lactation consultant. Score!

When my sister-in-law got to the house, she didn't even unpack her bags. She was on a mission, and within five minutes, she had my son latching on one side. Five minutes later, he was on the other side. I was stunned. These were my boobs, but she was getting them to do their thing. Like clockwork. Every four to five hours, she had that kid nursing. Just like that. To this day, I call her the "Nipple Whisperer."

Stick to what you feel is best for you and your baby. Ask for help. Beg for help. Call your sister-in-law. If you don't have one, borrow someone else's.

PUREE THIS

To this day, I still give my husband a hard time about how he said he wanted to puree the food for the baby. I looked up the definition of puree online. Here is what I found: "noun. a thick, moist, smooth-textured form of cooked vegetables, fruits, etc., usually made by pressing the pulp through a sieve or by whipping it in a blender."

That sounded like work. For years, I've seen these jars of baby food with cute cheeky babies on the labels. Just twist, turn, and serve. That sounds easy enough.

What food did we choose? Charles and I pretty much bought food that looked kinda like food we could stomach. But the smell can be hard to get past! If you're looking for recommendations, the sweet potato and banana are quite good!

SLEEP LIKE A BABY

There's a phrase, "Sleep like a baby." That may depend on which baby you're referring to. I can tell you that babies like to wake up during the night. A LOT. I really never got used to waking up to that wailing. It pretty much freaked me out because there was no warning—just bam, a very mad baby! You aren't even two months old, what do you have to be mad about? I would often wake up with this panic and think,

Whoa, what's that? Where am I? Who's crying? It was usually because he had wet his diaper or was hungry. Try not to fret—the cries sound much worse than the actual situation.

We maybe kinda-sorta did the "rock the baby to sleep" thing too long. But it worked. Until it didn't. He'd fall asleep if we rocked him, but would often wake right back up if we put him in his crib. We didn't let him cry himself to sleep until WE were crying ourselves to sleep.

CLIFFSNOTES, PLEASE

You've probably seen the books. They're yellow with black letters. They're called CliffsNotes. I loved the idea back in school. You could get the gist of a particular story without actually having to do all of the work. Genius!

Now I don't want to give the impression of being a slacker mom, but really the idea of knowing how things will turn out in life ahead of time would be awesome! And it's an abbreviated version, so you'll save time.

CliffsNotes for motherhood would be ideal. And each mom could have one just for her life. Think of it as a type of mother's helper. You can peek ahead to see what happens next.

Here is a sample of the type of information these CliffsNotes would include:

Yes, your baby is going to be colicky.

Your baby will go to sleep if you drive her around the block 50 times.

Yay! You will get that first grade teacher you hoped for.

That minivan you saw on Craigslist? Don't buy it.

Letting your child cry to sleep won't send her to therapy.

Your child will not get whooping cough, but he will get back-to-back ear infections within a two-month period.

The dog will love and protect your kids. The cat? Not so much.

The neighborhood kid with the tattoos and the body piercings is actually one of the best babysitters you'll find.

That four-bedroom ranch house you've been eyeing up has major plumbing issues.

Your husband is not cheating on you, but couples therapy would be a good idea.

The amount it will cost to raise your child from birth to 18 is four times the amount you calculated.

The bed that costs $2,500 could be one of the best investments for your back and your marriage.

Imagine all of the time, frustration, and money you could potentially save if you knew what was going to happen before it did. Sadly, there are no CliffsNotes for parenting. We figure out motherhood as we go along. But maybe some of the mothers before us could give us a heads-up now and then.

SAY SOMETHING. JUST NOT THAT

Alright. So the whole CliffsNotes thing isn't gonna happen. But there are so many times it would have been nice to get a heads-up.

Don't be surprised when your own family tells you what you don't want to hear. My friend made this great soup for our mom's group. She said it was super easy to make and gave me the recipe. This was mistake number one. Most days, dinner is almost like an after thought. By the time we get home from school, go through the back-packs, check the mail, do homework, and make a lunch for the next day, making dinner just doesn't seem like fun. How bad can it be to feed your kids cereal and chips for dinner?

My husband works later hours than me, and I'm always thinking how nice it would be to have a warm meal to come home to. So I made the soup just like my friend said. I thought anyway. Cream cheese, diced tomatoes, and tomato soup. I left her a message to call back and let me know what I may need to add.

When Charles got home and saw the soup on the stove, he asked, "What's that?"

Something in his tone told me he wasn't going to like it. When he sat down to eat the soup, he was sniffing it. Kinda like a dog does when you switch his food. Like, Hmm, what the hell is this stuff? Doesn't look like Dog Chow. They don't make Gravy Train anymore.

As Charles lifted the spoon to his mouth, he said, "You know it just looks like something, right?"

This was a statement not a question, so I didn't bother to comment. He began to eat the jailhouse slop, and then he said it again. "It just kinda looks like something, but I'm not gonna say anything." Oh, for Christ's sake, just say it already! Charles somehow managed to finish two bowls of the "stuff" and told me, "Please don't make that again. I mean, it looks like something. You know what it looks like, right?" No, honey, but you seem to really want to tell me what it looks like, I think.

"It looks like vomit." Then he turned the bowl so I could see the lumpy stuff with chunks of tomatoes. Actually, he was right. It had that barfed-up pizza look. And the sour smell from the cream cheese lended to the authenticity of it.

The phone rang. It's my friend.

"Julie, did you add a cup of water?" she asked.

"Too late," I told her.

I ruined it. Oh, and we had fun throwing it out. Charles slowly poured it into a paper bag while I made gagging sounds. I know, totally immature.

Well, at least now we know how to make vomit! I *am* good in the kitchen.

I'LL NEVER DO THAT. WHOOPS.

Daily there's a story in the news about what someone did and many people react saying things such as, "How could someone be so stupid?" I get it. Before I had kids, I thought the same way. Then I had kids, and I became stupid. I used to hear about parents who accidentally lock their infants in cars. That just seemed nearly impossible to do. But I managed that one. One day, my firstborn was about four months old and sound asleep in his infant carrier. What should have been a quick stop at Goodwill turned into 30 minutes of "Oh my God, Oh my God, Oh my God" with a steady stream of sweat to accompany it.

I got out to hand a bag of donated goods to an employee, and when I turned around to open the door, it was locked. The motor was running, and the heat was blasting on high. I could not have felt like a worse mother.

AAA was called, and the car was unlocked before the baby was even awake. That is one of the quickest ways to drop 5 pounds in one day.

YOU DON'T GET IT

You probably knew parenting wasn't going to be easy, but did you have any idea it would be this hard? It's like so many major life changes: marriage, divorce, career changes, and buying a house. You really don't know what it will be like until you are going through it. I always wanted to have a t-shirt with the slogan, "You don't know what you don't know until you know better."

For example, when we brought our son Miles home, I just couldn't believe how often we had to change his diapers. I kept thinking, How can such a tiny being fill so many diapers? And how can poop shoot all the way up his back?!

How could ladies breastfeed in public? I never understood that—until I had kids. It's not a peep show. There's no stripper pole or flashing of the breast. It comes down to two choices: a kid screaming so much he has area dogs covering their ears accompanied by a frenzied and lactating mom or a happy baby with a mom who isn't leaking through her bra. So yeah, who wouldn't feed on the go if they had the chance? Think of it as a mobile, maternal vending machine.

Of course we know how horrible fast food is. I was in the camp that swore our children would never eat fast food. I am not proud of the fact that they have frequented a certain fast food chain enough that they practically know the menu by heart! Dare I admit that I have allowed them eat that fat-laden food in front of the television, which of course some say is using an electronic device as a baby sitter. I'd rather call it mother's assistant. Legally, you have to pay a sitter.

Maybe you too judged those moms who used stern tones, a

few choice words, and a glare that would stop a cougar in his tracks while shopping with the kids. It's just shopping, right? Easy in. Easy out. Yes, when you don't have kids in tow. Otherwise not so much. The kids want to sit in the cart. The one that looks like a real truck. It might as well be registered with the DOT. Those things drive like a Mack Truck, and there's virtually no way to turn them around in the aisle. You have to back them up. All while little arms are reaching out, knocking things off the shelf. Two words: manager's nightmare.

All that's stuff we just didn't get—until we got it.

DON'T FORGET ABOUT YOU

5ks and 10ks are very popular these days. I was blown away by a Facebook status update from one of my friends. She had done a triathlon, including a half-mile swim, 14-mile bike ride, and 3.5-mile run. Under two hours. After a 20-year hiatus.

Hmmmm, 20 years ago, I was partying like a rock star. My diet consisted of Mountain Dew and cheap, greasy fast food. I smoked cigarettes, drank whiskey, and stayed up super late. Then I met my husband. Then I got pregnant. Twenty years later, I'm still trying to undo the rock-star-party damage plus all that stuff that happens to your body after having kids.

I'm not sure why my friend took a break from running and triathlons. But I know a lot of friends who took breaks because they had kids. It totally makes sense. But after staying home and watching Barney until you literally see purple, you want to go to a movie—at a theater with adults. After wearing clothes that are made almost completely of stretchy material, you want outfits that look fashionable and show off your waistline. After seemingly endless nights of rocking a wee one to sleep, we reserve the right to go to bed before the kids if we want.

You give up a lot when you have kids. But it was our choice. We signed up for it, even if we didn't read all the fine print. But that doesn't mean we should give up on doing the things we'd like to do. I'm thinking we and our kids are better off for it.

I commented on my friends' Facebook page saying I thought she was amazing. She wrote back inviting me to join her next year. I told her I'd skip all the sweaty stuff. Instead, I'd drive the whole distance and be done in 10 minutes. That would give me one hour and 50 minutes to check out a movie and meet her at the finish line!

DON'T FORGET YOUR BABY DADDY

"Everything's always about the kids!" That's something my husband says often.

If you take a look around at who and what was in your life

before children, it might be different after they come along. Not to say that kids are relationship wreckers. But they rely on us as parents so much, and after a while it kind of seems like we're codependent on that. Life becomes a preemptive move to serve the baby this, and get the kids that. Meanwhile your husband or partner feels left out—although cable television will help keep him occupied, he needs more.

But truly it can be difficult to find a way to make everyone happy. Okay, it's maybe even impossible as someone will likely cry. But it is important to keep your adult relationships intact.

Even though date night sounds wonderful, the idea of leaving an infant in someone else's care can make you panic. But here's a thought. If you go away for a few hours, the baby won't recall that and there will be no harm done. If you neglect your husband, it will come up in every fight you'll ever have.

You deserve a break. And it can be something simple like going for a scenic walk or window shopping at the mall. Or sit at someone else's house and watch *their* cable TV. Together.

BABY NUMBER TWO

When your doctor tells you can get pregnant while breastfeeding, believe them. And believe me.

PSST, ARE YOU AWAKE?

After having children, sleep is hard to come by. I remember waking up as a kid and realizing that my parents had been up for hours. It never made sense to me. I was thinking, *Why are they up so early? How boring.*

Fast forward 30-some years, and I get it. The moment you have a baby, you sign up for sleep deprivation. Forever. Even though the baby eventually sleeps through the night, you might not.

The *New York Times* reported that more mothers are using prescription pills to help get sleep. You would think as exhausted as we can get, it would be easy to fall asleep. Most of us are busy trying to keep it together. Stay-at-home moms are on call 24/7. Moms who work outside the home go from one job to another.

But even once you are in bed, the noise in your head continues. What was the RSVP date for the wedding? Where is the RSVP card for the wedding? Can I get a sitter that night? I hope I can find her cell number. When can I get to the store to buy them a gift? Wait, where are they registered again? And a card. I gotta get a card. And a new dress. Or maybe I can just wear something I have.

Sadly, alcohol doesn't help. A few weeks ago, I had a Mojito (or two) that had me falling fast asleep. Until 3 am. There I was, no more buzz and no more sleep.

Sleeping-in rarely happens. Even when I *do* sleep until 6 am, I feel a panic of, *Wait, how come I slept so late? Did I oversleep? What am I supposed to be doing?*

So yeah, it's no wonder moms are having a hard time falling to sleep. Life is a constant merry-go-round, and it won't slow down. I don't even like those things at the fair.

Think of all the times you've chatted with a friend who told you she was up all night. And you replied, "Me too. You should have called me." So I'm thinking we could have a hotline. When you can't sleep, you dial in. We could chat about our days, our kids, our spouses. We could exchange recipes and share decorating ideas. We would be able to network and provide tips on parenting, job hunting, and coupon clipping. There's only one problem. We'd be awake.

Goodnight.

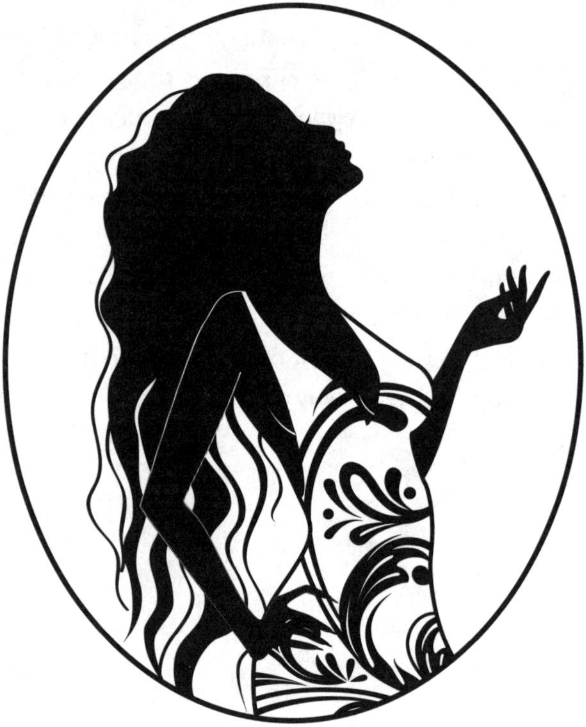

6

Older and Wiser

UMMM... THANKS FOR THE HONESTY

One evening, our son Miles found me in the kitchen and asked if he could look at our wedding pictures.

After taking a look, he said, "I think Mommy should look like she used to in the wedding pictures."

I try to mentally prepare myself before asking, "And how did I used to look?"

Of course, he had an answer.

"Well, you used to be thin. And you used to be tall and straight. "

What the? Okay, yes I was 40 pounds lighter when we got married, but God don't tell me I'm crooked now too!

I looked at Charles for some type of support. Help me out, man! He quickly looked up from his laptop and said, "You're shrinking."

Then he went right back to his computer. Just like that. Thank you, Judas, nice to see you too! And what is this used to be "straight" crap? Like I'm bent. But before I could question that, my son continued his list of "How Mommy used to be." "And you had smooth skin, no pimples."

I don't have pimples (much)! Ugh! I turned to go back to the kitchen. But I heard my son telling Charles, "Daddy, I saw this commercial on TV for something that would make Mommy's pimples go away. It would make her skin pretty again. I say pretty because I'm not supposed to say sexy."

Let's sum this up, shall we. I'm increasing in width, decreasing in height, and pimples are taking over. It's best to know when you are outnumbered and just take your crooked butt to bed.

BATHROOM HUMOR

I felt I must add a disclaimer here. If you don't like to hear about poop, bottoms, or penises, then you might want to skip this section. I have boys, and for some reason there's almost daily discussion about poop. But if that turns you off, perhaps you will want to move on to the entry titled "What's in Your Boobs?" It's silly and fun. And there's no mention of poop.

GOTTA FIND THAT BUTT HOLE

Just one week before my youngest son's fifth birthday, he discovered there's a hole in his bottom. And he wanted to see it!

I was in my room, and I heard someone moving around in the bathroom. After I made my way there, I found my son completely naked, grabbing his butt cheeks and pulling them apart—all while he was stretching his neck to look over his shoulder to get a peek at this new-found body part. But it wasn't working. Instead, his body was twisted, and he kept turning around and around like a dog chasing his tail!

At this point, I was thinking that he will realize that he just won't be able to get a look at the hole in his butt. Nope. He's got a plan B. Now he's on the floor on his back, lifting his knees up to look between his legs. Man, he was determined. But again, he wasn't having much luck, and he looked like a very small, naked break dancer. You could almost hear him asking "Where IS that stink hole?"

I totally understand that curiosity is normal, but I couldn't help but wonder about something else. What happens when he discovers the appendage on the front of his body?

WAIT! YOU HAVE A BUTT HOLE TOO?

Sometimes I wonder: What if I have a day where there's nothing to write? I mean, I don't need to be comical all the time. I can write about serious stuff, but still, what if there's a day of "nothing"? No fits, no fights. Nothing.

Then, just as I cleaned up the morning breakfast mess, I heard my husband yelling from the bathroom "That is so disgusting! You could get kicked out of the family for that. For sure kicked out of school!" Did he say "kicked out of the family?" Oooh, this is gonna be good! As I headed upstairs, I saw Charles. He was at the top of the steps, and he was so mad he was huffing.

"They are looking at each other's butt holes!" he angrily told me.

I know it was wrong, like really, really wrong, but all I could do was laugh.

My mind went back to when our younger son was naked in the bathroom holding his butt cheeks, trying to see his new-found anus. He wore himself out spinning around and around trying to get a look at it. I mean hey, why not see if your brother has one too? 'Cause wouldn't it suck to find out you were the only one in the family with a butt hole? Or worse yet, the only one *without* one!

MOM, THE TRAFFIC CONTROLLER

Like many mothers, I chose to stay home with my children for a few years and then return to working outside the home. The problem is that after staying home for a while, there's a gap in the resume.

Moms need to take a hard look at all they do. The list is endless: launderer, referee, chef, chauffeur, counselor, triage nurse. Where am I going with this? Not sure you even want to know, but since I'm this far into it, I'm adding traffic controller to my list of duties and responsibilities. Most often, this traffic directing takes place in the bathroom.

Eleven years ago, my husband and I bought our current house. We convinced ourselves it was an upgrade from our previous home. First, we no longer had to take a ladder to the outside of the house in spring and fall to change the storm windows. That required more dexterity and physical strength than we signed up for. And there was generally a bit of cussing involved.

The second thing we now have is central air. Ahhhhh....cold air right here in our house. We don't have to sit through awful movies or wander around in circles in department stores to soak up their AC. We've got our own.

But what we didn't think through was the fact that our house is a "one holer." Yes. A house with one bathroom. I think this didn't occur to us as a problem when we bought the house because at the time, the boys weren't completely potty trained. But still, what were we thinking? That they'd stay in diapers into adulthood? I believe it was more, Oh we could totally put a toilet in the basement. No problem.

Here's the rub. There are 24 hours in a day. We have four toilet-using people in the house. This gives each of each six hours of time to use the bathroom. Yet every morning without fail, everyone needs to use the toilet—at the same time!

Here's how this works.

"I gotta go...bad!"

"Sorry, you should have woke up earlier."

"You've been in there 20 minutes!"

"Have not."

"Have to."

Enter Mom, the traffic controller.

"Okay, get up. Let your brother go."

"I'm pooping!"

"Have you actually pooped yet?

"No, but I'm trying,"

"And you. Do you need to go number one or number two?"

"Number one."

Okay. Get up for 10 seconds and let your brother pee!"

"Not fair!"

"No, it's not. But get up because there's a line."

"That's okay, Mom. Can I just go in the sink?"

"WHAT? For the love of...just go while your brother takes a quick break!"

"Thanks. You can sit back down."

And just when all should be well.

"He peed on the seat!"

They still sell ice cream in those gallon buckets, right? Hmmm. I think I could use one or two of those. Perfect. I can add problem solver to my resume too.

DON'T SCRATCH THAT ITCH

No matter how organized you might be, the morning routine is hectic. No one wants to get up. Somebody doesn't like the clothing selection. Everybody is tired. And sometimes somebody gets "itchy."

I found my son in his room kind of wiggling against his bed. I asked him what was wrong. "My butt itches," he told me.

"Okay, hold on," I said as I headed to the bathroom for a washcloth.

"Here honey," I called out to him.

He didn't meet me in the bathroom, so I headed back to his room.

Tell me this is not happening. He is sitting on the floor, scooting himself forward as he drags his butt across the carpet! If you have a dog, you have witnessed the four-legged version of this.

I didn't know whether to laugh or cry. I mean when you got an itch...

On the other hand, I know that this cannot have a happy ending. Either he will have carpet fuzz in his butt or...

Yep. We should have gone with the dark shag carpet!

DO ALL GIRLS HAVE THOSE?

I try to make privacy a top priority at our house. Especially when it comes to the bathroom. Inevitably, sometimes I find what seems like the perfect moment to use the bathroom but am interrupted by one of the kids.

Such was the case in this situation. My younger son burst into the room and said, "I really gotta go!" I don't get that. He's gone like 10 hours, and now he's gotta get in here?

"Okay, but give me some privacy. I'll be right out," I said.

He turned to leave but then backed up and gave me this bewildered look. Oh, boy. I could feel one of those awkward questions coming.

He's looking toward my back end and says, "It's weird that you pee out of your butt."

"What? I don't pee..." Then it dawns on me that he is not aware of the female anatomy and assumes that because I am sitting down that I must be peeing from my butt.

I explained to him that boys have different private parts than girls. I felt so grown up. I even said the word "vagina." Before that, I worried he'd tell everyone he met that his mom has one. Or maybe yell it down the halls at school.

As he walked out of the bathroom he looked at me in

disbelief and said, "That's just weird." *You don't know the half of it, kid,* I thought.

So that night while my son was brushing his teeth, he called me into the bathroom. He looked up at me with his toothbrush to one side of his mouth. There was that inquisitive look again as he asked, "Mom, do girl kids have those 'chinas' too?"

It was late, and you know, he was six. Who cares if he has the name wrong? Plus, how much trouble can he get in at school for yelling "china"?

"Yes, honey, girl kids have chinas too."

WHAT'S IN YOUR BOOBS?

I think it's a bit disturbing to say that a little boy will grow up to be a "leg man" or "boob man." First, they are not men; they're little boys. Second, it sounds like how you would describe chicken parts you want with the butcher.

Having said that, I wonder if men take an interest in certain female parts at an early age. My younger son seems fascinated with boobs.

"Mom, what's in your boobs?" he asked me in a curious tone.

I was so shocked, I initially didn't answer. Then, not knowing how to answer, I asked him, "What do you mean what's in them?"

"Like on the inside. Is it blood and veins?"

I thought for a bit before I answered. I really wasn't sure what was in them, but I wanted to sound like I did.

"Well, mostly they have fat tissue in them."

That seemed to satisfy him. For a few days.

And then there were more questions.

"Do girls have to have boobs?"

Now that was one I could answer.

"Yep. Girls are born with them."

By now his little mind was really working on figuring this boob stuff out.

"Well, what happened to the milk that was in there before?"

Okay, the whole conversation was getting a little old to me, so I looked him square in the face and said, "It dried up, and there is no more."

He seemed satisfied with that answer.

As I began writing this entry, my son came over and gave me a hug. And something dawned on me. From infancy, we cradle our kids and pull them to our chest as we comfort them. As they get older, it's the same thing. When they need comfort, we bring them to our chest.

I'm not saying that we should bring them to our butts or legs, but perhaps that is why so many guys are fixated with our chests. Warm, soft, and squishy; maybe a pillow would be useful instead.

GREY: IT'S THE NEW BROWN

Something about having children ages us. I don't mind the actual turning one year older, but the physical changes. Like grey hair. Except for Michael McDonald, who looks good with all that grey? As my hair dresser said, "You have those angry grey hairs." Much like foil.

Try pulling those buggers out. It's like trying to pull those thistle weeds from your garden. You can pull them so far out, but you can still see them near the root.

WHY MUST THEY USE FOUR-POINT TYPE?

The past few years, I started thinking I need bifocals. When I read, I have to adjust my arm length from my body like three times. Yet, my eyes were fine just a few months ago.

A few years ago, I called an optometrist to get some answers. He asked my age. I told him 42. He said (without hesitation mind you),"Yep. You're at *that* age. That's all." That's all? Dude, my eyesight was 20/20, and then "Bam" everything's blurry. That's *all*?

But at 40 (here we go again), things looked dirty. I could see people, but reading became a chore. I would rub my eyes, squint, and move my arm near and far until I got just the right distance to read.

I'm pretty sure the tipping point was when I gave my son Miles too much medicine. I'm not even sure what medicine it was, but I couldn't read the dosage line on the dispenser right.

Not to justify my mistake, but I suggest those dosage markers be marked in black. Most of the time, they are simply etched in the plastic. It's like Braille, only not the kind that anyone is familiar with.

So after a frantic call to Poison Control, I decided maybe I should have my eyes looked at. I had gone to the optometrist one year earlier and never filled my prescription. I left with no intent on returning.

So I humbly went back to the eye doctor and found out that I did, in fact, need glasses. This turned out to be much more complicated than I thought. Did I want the anti-glare lenses? What? So other people don't stare at me? Sorry, but this was new territory for me.

It turns out that I needed bifocals. That truly made me feel old. Then the assistant asked if I wanted the kind with or without the line on the lens. For the love of Pete, I'm 42 years old, why would I want to advertise my advanced age by way of that horrible line on my glasses?

I was feeling overwhelmed and not in the mood for this new not-so-cool accessory. As horrible as this sounds, I kept thinking, *No one with glasses is sexy. Okay good looking. Maybe. But not sexy.* Which is hilarious because I'm not sexy now! But getting these glasses made me feel even less so.

I saw a poster in the office of a very attractive woman wearing glasses. I was not convinced one bit. She was simply a model who wore the glasses for the photo shoot only. I imagined that after an hour's worth of posing, she whipped off those glasses, relieved that she didn't have to wear them for real.

It just bothered me. I was trying to imagine strippers with glasses. Not a chance. Then it dawned on me that there had to be a ton of ladies who had poor eyesight but who wore contacts. As immature as this might be, that thought gave me great relief. Now I could see myself as a sexy lady who *chose* to wear glasses.

After an exhaustive search, one of the ladies on staff found a frame that was perfect. It had some bling on it, and on the side, I saw Harley Davidson. Oh yeeeaahhh, a biker babe with glasses! I was good to go.

Though I was a bit tempted, I had to walk away from the things that attach to your glasses and you wear around your neck. No way, no how is that sexy. So I kept on walking.

WHAT'S THAT CLICKING SOUND?

My knees have begun to make this clicking sound, so I talked with my doctor about it.

"It's likely arthritis," he said. "Unfortunately, it comes with age."

Here we go again. It comes with age? Like something on a menu. "That comes with fries or cole slaw." Who ordered it? I didn't!

I guess I would have liked a heads up, you know. Maybe like a public service announcement. "This is a friendly reminder that your body will most certainly fall apart between 40 and 45. This may include, but is not limited to, menopause, mood swings, absent mindedness, decreased hearing, poor eyesight, and crackling knees. You may seek medical attention, but really not much can be done. Do not yell at your doctor. It is not her fault. You're aging, and possibly you got bad genes."

Since I'm adopted, a note would have been nice. Maybe, "We wish you well and hope you enjoy your new family. Oh, and sorry about the bad-knee thing, kid."

Then I realize that I tell my boys that age doesn't define them. I tell them, "It doesn't matter that you are young; there are lots of things you can do." So, I guess that I should go by the same idea—that my age doesn't define me. Okay, fine.

I'm happy to report that the leg brace I bought is helping with the knee thing. Plus it gives me sympathy at the gym and around the office. And I suppose I could see that glasses could be seen as a cool accessory. But I'm not gonna stop coloring my hair. No way, no how.

IT'S NOT A FAIRY TALE

The upside of aging is that it's accompanied with maturity. Like realizing that how we thought it was gonna be—isn't.

After 72 days, Kim Kardashian found out that she no longer wanted to be married to Kris Humphries. She told *Glamour* magazine, "It means that I believe in love and the dream of having a perfect relationship, but my idea of it has changed. I think I need to not live in a fairy tale like that. I think I maybe need to just snap out of it and be a little more realistic."

As young girls, we might have had some fairy tale thoughts, but as most of us found out, that's just not realistic. And really that isn't all bad.

For one thing, fairy tales have knights in white armor. Think about that get-up. Very cold. Not to mention out of date. My guy wears Levi's.

Or Prince Charming. If he's so charming, how come he was never married before?

If you live in a fairy tale, you wear poofy dresses. Can you imagine nursing a kid in that type of outfit? Oh, and there is a crown. It does look a bit pretentious.

A fully loaded minivan is way cooler and faster than a horse-drawn carriage. That's not gonna work shuttling kids to violin lessons and soccer games.

In fairy tales, there are fairies everywhere. And they

carry dust. Like we don't have enough to clean up already!

And pardon me for saying this: Gnomes are creepy.

Characters in the fairy tale world live in castles. Do you know how much it would cost to heat that thing?

Fairy tales are great. For Disney. For the rest of us, maybe a minivan, a husband with a slight beer belly, and imperfect kids are just fine. Maybe maids waiting on us every now and then would be okay though.

IS IT HOT IN HERE?

Then there is the part of life that is truer than we would like. Enter the wonderful change in life.

A few months ago, I woke up in the middle of the night. I was hot. Like burning from the inside out hot. Like I'd been working out hot. But I hadn't been working out. I had been enjoying deep sleep until I was so rudely awakened by my hotness. No, unfortunately not hotness like Beyoncé or Kate Moss. I'm talking flushed, damp, sweaty hot. Nice visual, huh?

Looking for relief, I kicked off the sheets. No relief there. I turned on the fan. Still hot. Finally, convinced that I had a fever, I dragged my butt out of bed and took my temperature. Exactly 98.6 degrees.

Then I couldn't sleep, so I did what any wide awake gotta-know-what-is-wrong-with-me-now wife would do. I got back in bed and drove my husband crazy.

"Is it warm in here? Do you think the heat is too high?" I asked, waking him up from what was probably a perfectly good night's sleep. I kept placing my hand on his back, checking to see if he had any cool spots.

Ahhh, he feels perfect, I thought.

At some point, it was suggested that I was having a hot flash. Hot flash? Oh, man. Those are reserved for ladies going through menopause, right? I've got young kids. I couldn't be going through menopause. I simply don't have the time. You know? I have more important things to do.

So the next day, still reeling from the "hot" episode, I decided to get to the bottom of things. Yeah, I should have called the doctor. Instead, I Googled "symptoms of menopause." Holy....I couldn't believe it. I'm thinking there's gonna be like five symptoms. Wrong. The list I found had 35 symptoms. That's five plus 30! I thought that my sweaty legs (or "swegs" as the young interns at work hipped me to) were bad. This list had things I'd never imagined, like "changes in fingernails, itchy, crawly, skin." How about "disturbing memory lapses and dry vagina." Dry vagina? Oh, but that's okay, I might work that out via the "increased incontinence."

Obviously, I made a wrong turn by searching the web. But I do remember after giving birth feeling like I could do anything. I'm praying there's a kernel of truth to that, because if this menopause list is even close to accurate, I'm expecting everything!

Itchy. Crawly. Skin. Really?

SCOOT, MOM, SCOOT!

At some point, to get your old body back, you might choose to work out. Remember how easy it was to lose those pounds after having babies? Yeah, me neither. And though my older son is well meaning, it doesn't help that he is a total believer of every commercial he sees.

"Hey, Mom, look at this commercial! You can lose 10 pounds in two weeks. Is that what you need?"

Admittedly, I was embarrassed to start running. It really isn't a good visual. In my younger years, I had this great stride and was carefree. Now I take small steps. I'm nervous to step on something the wrong way and twist my ankle. I imagine my neighbors watching me from inside their homes and trying to describe what they see.

"No, honey, she's not running. It's more like a scoot."

But it's cool because I found that there's this sort of runner's respect other runner's show me now. Sort of like Harley riders. Without the motorcycle. And without the leather gear. Okay, okay. What I mean is that other runners

(I mean the ones that are really running, the non-scooters) make a point to give me a nod or say hello. And whenever another runner acknowledges me, all I can think is, *Cool! They think I'm one of them!*

During one of my runs, three women were running in my direction. They were laughing and carrying on. There I was, hardly able to keep a steady breath, let alone speak. Then one of them gave me a smile and a wave. As much as I was ready to stop my run for the day I waited 'til they were out of my view before I came to a halt. I didn't want them thinking they'd wasted a wave and a hello on some second rate runner.

But what is really nice is the kids want to join me. They like to ride their bikes while Mommy scoots behind them. Seeing as how I am unable to run and speak at the same time, I came up with hand signals for stop, slow down, and keep going. I probably need one for "Mommy needs oxygen," but I think they'll figure that one out.

SO WE LOOK A LITTLE DIFFERENT

I came across a study that said 33 percent of wives think that their husbands find them less attractive since having kids. And the majority of the women said they felt tired.

Then I got to thinking, maybe we aren't less attractive.

Maybe we just don't place the same amount of emphasis on our attractiveness as we used to. And quite possibly that is because we are tired.

Just when I have rationalized all this attractiveness stuff, my oldest son remarks, "Not to be mean, Mom, but how come you aren't as pretty as you were when you were younger?"

Well, let's see. I didn't have a job that I cared if I lost or kept so there was no stress on the work front. Happy hour wasn't when an infant went to sleep. It was cheap drinks and laughs with my pals from the office. My metabolism actually worked. There was no need for coloring my hair. There were none of those grey imposters working their way in. I basically really only had to worry about me. No worrying meant I could sleep uninterrupted for hours! I was free to go places besides Target.

I didn't want to tell him those things. It was a harmless question. And truthfully, I signed up for this life. Well, except for the stretch marks. I just kind of shrugged it off and vaguely explained that people change when they get old.

Later that same day, my younger son and I were face-to-face discussing something. At one point, he stopped talking to me and reached out to touch my face. His right index finger landed smack dab in between my eyes.

"Why do you have lines there?"

Sigh. I asked my husband about the fact that my appearance has changed since having kids. He said he constantly tells me he thinks I'm attractive, but that I don't listen. Note to self: Start listening. And if it's good stuff, believe it!

WE'VE BECOME OUR PARENTS

I recall thinking that my parents just didn't get it. Or they didn't get me. Oh, how I was sadly mistaken. It didn't take much more than five minutes of parenting to realize that.

To a kid, it's like your parents are speaking a different language. Think of all those crazy things they said. Here were some of my favorites.

"Stop crying before I give you something to cry about." Okay, let's investigate this. We were already crying for whatever reason and now our parents were going to find another reason to cry. Does that make any sense? I was already crying, for Pete's sake!

But think about it with your own kids. There are just times when you've had it with the whining and crying. Really. All they have to do is get up, eat the food we prepared, and share their toys. How hard can that be? Very. And that's when we tell them that we have a list of threats we can arbitrarily hand out to get the tears rolling.

"Because I said so!" Man, that one was so unfair. Just like that, we as kids had to go along with the plan just because our parents told us to? There was no wiggle room. Nor room for discussion. Now, as a parent, you can see how convenient this statement is. It's a one-size-fits-all excuse. At the end of a long day when your brain is fried, you no longer have to make sense. Why? Because you said so!

"Just wait until you have kids of your own!" What a cheap shot! First, it made it seem like our parents didn't really want us, as if we were a burden. And that statement was no different than telling us, "Payback is a bitch." But in your quest to get your kids to "get it," it may be one of the first things that flies out of your mouth. If you think back, you actually had a response to this one, but because you valued your life, you didn't dare speak it. That response would have been, "Yeah, well I won't be a mean parent like you." Yep. And then you find yourself that mean parent.

"My house, my rules." Ring a bell? Totally unfair when you were a kid. Kids can't own homes. So there you were counting down the days until you were an adult and could buy a house. Then you'd invite your parents over and make them adhere to your rules. Now there's poetic justice! So be leery when your kids ask you to stop by.

Yeah our parents were clueless. They told us ridiculous things. They made no sense. Now, we get to carry on the tradition of spewing clichés to our own kids in hopes they won't realize these borrowed words were the same ones we swore we'd never repeat. Eh, do as I say, not as I do.

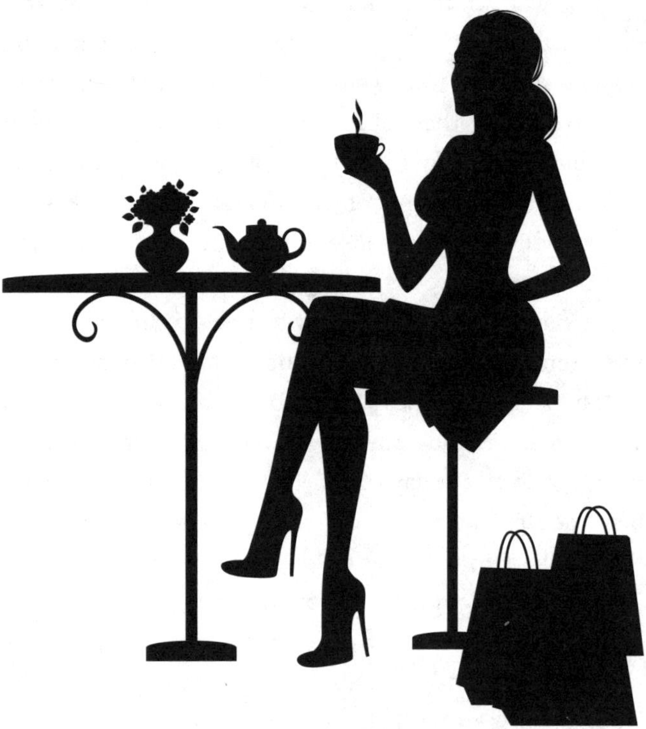

7

Mom My Time

NOW I GET IT

You might have read about the family that called 911 from a corn maze. They had a newborn and a five year old with them, and they panicked when they couldn't find their way out. My first thought was, *C'mon, how can you get lost in a corn maze?*

The week after, we met some other families for an afternoon of fun in a corn maze. Before we ventured into the maze, the staff showed us a video and a map of the corn maze. Then they went over the rules. Rule number two was no foul language. That should have been my first clue that this was not for me. I can safely say that after two hours of wandering through a corn maze, with hungry kids, as the cold and darkness settled in, while trying not to use inappropriate language, I can totally see how you might be tempted to call 911. They would have easily found me. Follow the voice of the mom using foul language bribing her kids with Happy Meal, and shouting "How the Hell do we get outta here?"

PHONE A FRIEND, AGAIN!

One of the best ways to decompress is by connecting with friends. Someone who also "gets" what you are going through. Maybe it's that "misery loves company" thing. Or maybe we just need a place to vent and know that no one will judge us for complaining about what we signed up for.

Once children enter the picture, it's not so easy to get together with friends. Nap schedules, stomach flus, availability of babysitters, and overdrawn checking accounts have a way of limiting your social life.

Thank goodness for telephones. But beware: As soon as you start a good conversation, the chaos starts. It's amazing that no one seems to notice you until you pick up the phone. Just as you're getting into some good gossip, pouring out your heart and soul, or lamenting about what feels like the worst day ever, someone has a major meltdown. It makes no sense. They'll seem perfectly content playing on the Wii or doing an art project. You don't even exist. Until you start that phone conversation. Then it's total mayhem. Someone won't share their toys. Someone else can't find that one critical piece from the 400-piece Lego set.

So often times you have these conversations with a friend that repeats itself. "I'm sorry. Can you hold on? The kids keep talking to me." Then you go from being mild mannered to screaming, "Can't you see I'm on the phone?!"

The conversation goes on and on this way until you've had enough and hang up to deal with the youngins who have been pulling the shenanigans in the first place. Guess what happens the moment you put the phone down?

It's tempting to pick up the phone again, but if the thought tires you out, try emailing a friend.

DO MOMS REALLY READ THIS STUFF?

One way to connect with other women is to join a group of some sort. Like a book club. A while back, I was thrilled to be asked to join one. Not because I like reading. Seriously, I still like picture books. But this group of women is really cool. So when they asked if I wanted to join, I was all over it.

The month one of my friends was hosting book club, she sent out an e-mail about the book she wanted us to read. She said the book had cussing. And crime. And sex. Great, now our husbands might want to join. The title of the book was G *Spot*. Gulp.

So there I was, wondering how I was gonna get the book. The library? It would be my luck to get to the check-out and realize my card was expired. Meanwhile, the librarian would have the book on the counter in plain sight while she updated my card. And I could see her giving me quick looks of disapproval, calling me a pervert in her mind.

If I ordered the book in the mail, it would get delivered while I was at work. It wouldn't fit in the mail slot, so the delivery person would take it to my neighbor's house next door. Then I'd have to get it from her, and before she'd hand it over to me she'd undoubtedly ask what it is. I can imagine the conversation now. "Oh that looks like a book. What's the title?" She's a huge reader, so lying isn't really an option, so I'd tell her. *"It's called G Spot."*

Then there would be this awkward 10-second pause before I'd tell her it's a gag gift for a bachelorette party. Then she'd smile and tell me that it sounds like the perfect raunchy gift for such an occasion.

Whatever. I decided I would just go to Barnes and Noble after church on Sunday. Yeah. I'll ask for forgiveness, and then get to sinning.

There we were, kids in tow at the bookstore. Charles told me to get the book. I reminded him of the title, and he quickly took the boys to the kids' section. Okay that part is taken care of. I really don't need the boys saying, "Hey how come the lady on the cover is kind of naked? I see boobs."

I had no clue where to find the book, so I headed to the check-out I usually go to. Great. It's a guy. I suddenly felt really dirty.

"Um, do you have the book *G Spot?*" I asked.

"The name is *G Spot?*" he asked.

Oh, God. I should have gone the mail order route.

"Yes, that's the title."

He got on his computer, and I'm standing there beginning to get flushed. It was worse than waiting to see if you have exceeded your credit limit as you make a purchase.

He looked up from his computer and pointed to another counter that I need to go to. Then he got on his walkie-talkie thing and said, "Customer assistance lower level." He said something else that I didn't understand, and I was convinced that it was code for "dirty book purchase." Perfect. Now all of the employees can look at the 40-something lady who's buying the steamy read.

As I headed over to the "dirty book" counter, I saw an older couple heading over too. I walked slowly, hoping they would go ahead of me, but they motioned for me to go first. I met the new customer service guy. I really didn't want to have to say the name of the book. It's like a drug deal or something.

The best I could muster was, "I was told you could find a book for me."

He gave me a look like he wanted to say, "Yeah. That's what we do here. We sell people books."

He didn't say that, but he did ask me the name of the book. Oh no. And the old people were behind me.

"*G Spot*." I said. He looked up at me like he doesn't understand me.

"I'm sorry. Say again?" He asked.

On top of being embarrassed, I was getting upset.

Say again? No I don't want to say it again! Give me the book! I thought to myself.

"It's called *G Spot*," I very curtly replied.

He began typing away on his computer.

"It looks like we have a copy," he said. "You need to go back to that other counter."

What the...? Aren't they paid to get books for people? Oh I get it. If you want a "dirty book," you have to get it yourself. Like bagging your own groceries at the discount grocery stores.

So five minutes into my smut book journey, I'm back where I started. Now the first guy to help me saw me at the counter and turned to the shelf behind him. I feel very dirty. Not to mention my kids are in the same store.

At this point, I had very little dignity left. "Is the book back there behind the counter because it's dirty?" I asked the guy.

He told me no. He explained that they changed the store around and had to move inventory. That helped salvage some of my self-respect.

So joining a book club might add to your social circle. But I kept feeling that as a mom, I shouldn't be reading that kind of stuff. Ridiculous. I know. But I will say searching for, buying, and reading a Dr. Seuss book was far less stressful.

MAKE NEW FRIENDS, BUT KEEP THE OLD...

I know plenty of women who don't have mothers to turn to for help in their own role as a mom. For some, their moms are deceased. For others, the relationship is strained at best. Or sadly their moms just weren't there for them. Divorce, addiction, abandonment, and abuse typically have an ill effect on us as kids. And that spills over to adulthood.

My own mother died when I was 20. She never saw me graduate from college, get married, or have kids. For a while, I was angry. Angry that she was no longer here. Angry that my friends still had mothers. Angry that I had to do so much without her. I felt that I got ripped off. But after a while, that angry stuff gets old. Plus, my mom taught me that good can come from bad.

One night when Max was seven years old, I tucked him into bed and told him, "Your grandmother would have loved to have met you. I'm sad she isn't here."

In a very sleepy voice, he asked, "Yeah, but now you have kids to make you happy, right?"

Enough said.

The other thing that had really been resounding in my mother's absence is the circle of women I have around me. I have found strength, nurturing, and guidance from many women in my life. Until having children, I didn't even realize how important that would be. Here are some favorites in my life.

Sisters-in-law. They're like sisters, but without the childhood baggage. There's no bad feelings about which one of you was the favorite daughter. Your brothers might be sick of you, but you get to start fresh with their wives. Since they are in the family, they understand some of the history and antics of your family.

Daycare workers. They are working the front lines and will give it to you straight. They have seen countless women stressed out over working outside the home, wrought with guilt about not being with their wee ones most of the day. They get it.

Friends. If you can't turn to your friends for consolation, it might be time to get new ones. Seriously, most of your friends should be there to get you through trying times. Obviously, the ones who also have kids are great to commiserate with. Misery truly does love company.

But don't discount the friends who don't have kids. Truthfully, just because you have kids doesn't mean you're a good parent. Some of the best advice I've gotten has been from friends who don't have children. For some reason, they don't waffle on decision making, and they have direct advice. It's as if they have more clarity from the outside looking in. The rest of us are wallowing in a haze of wishy washyness, where we often fail to look at our situation from all perspectives.

Play groups. When I was young, my parents just opened up the back door and off we went. Now it's all about scheduled play time.

Our oldest son, Miles, was 15 months old, and I was 7

months pregnant when I read about a local play group. I hesitated before going. Hemmed and hawed. I kept thinking, *Why would I need a place like that?* I convinced myself that it wouldn't be worth my time. But then I got sick of watching *Thomas the Tank Engine*, *Blues Clues*, and *Dora the Explorer*.

So I went. What do you know? There was a room full of women who could relate to what I was going through. New moms, pregnant moms, moms who stayed at home, moms who worked outside the home. We talked about breastfeeding, diapers, toys, and food. And we shared our other passions—writing, cooking, and music.

That was 13 years ago. They were then total strangers, and now they're some of my best friends. We have seen each other through illness, divorce, weight loss, and job changes. Play groups can be more important to the adults than to the kids. Now we get together without the kids and sippy cups. It's adults only and cocktails!

The pool, the park, and the grocery store are filled with women who might be experiencing the same things as you. My husband is always saying I talk too much. That might be true, but connecting to other moms is vital. It comes down to realizing that other ladies are dealing with the same issues as you. And that means you aren't a weirdo. And even if you are weird, you're in the company of other like-minded weird people. Validation should never be underestimated.

MOM'S GOTTA HAVE FUN TOO

There are people you connect with. And for different reasons. Usually you have something in common. Maybe you met in college. Or you see each other at the dog park. Or it's the one person at work who doesn't make you wish you'd quit your job. When you send the kids off to school, you add to that social network.

It's interesting to see those relationships evolve. I look back as a mom of a k5er (no, it's not a word, but it works) and see how things were. We had difficulty remembering each other's names. We often just referred to people as, "that one kid's mom." We were nervous parents, worried if our kids would learn their ABCs and share their toys. Most of our conversations were in passing in the hallways or parking lot.

Fast forward seven years. Same parents. Same kids. Different dynamics. We used to set up play dates with the kids. We've learned it's just as important to set up dates *without* the kids.

Recently I went to a birthday party for one of the other moms. Yeah. Just a little different. Instead of rushing to our cars like we do for the morning drop-off, we rushed to give each other those big oh-my-goodness-I-can-hardly-breathe kinda hugs. We told our kids to not run around at restaurants. That night we had our own dance floor going!

Our kids have been told that alcohol isn't what it's

cracked up to be. After having my fill of adult beverages, I heard someone say it was time to do shots. Nope, not the kind for the flu.

When we first met, our conversations were limited to the niceties like how our kids were doing in school and would we be going to the fall dance. Now we share deeper stuff. Like divorce. Job loss. Frustration with trying to be the best parent possible. It's grown-up stuff.

It's ironic that we want our kids to make friends. But along the way, we do too.

Be open to invitations and keep your adult sippy cup handy. "That one kid's mom" could be your lifeline, dance partner, and friend all in one.

SEXY HAS A WHOLE NEW MEANING

Okay, so sexy is one of those subjective words. But I think in the dictionary it should read like this: Adjective "of, or pertaining to being and feeling attractive in a sexual manner to the opposite sex." I kind of threw up a little in my mouth too.

In the mother's post-kids dictionary, it might read something like this: "Of or pertaining to anything that is comfortable, oversized, and does not show stretch marks."

Look, I'm not trying to get picked up at a bar or anything, but when do you go from the hot pink underwear to the granny pants? I still have a pair of thong underwear from before we were married, and every time I look at them I think of how wearing them will make me feel like I have a piece of cloth stuck in between my butt cheeks.

Do you ever walk past Victoria's Secret and roll your eyes? Me too! Yeah, we know your secret, Victoria. You haven't gone through nine months of pregnancy and hard labor. Or breastfeeding. You cater to the 20-somethings who still have flat stomachs, perky breasts, and hips that have no idea how far they can spread. Your bras and underwear are not compatible with maxi pads with wings, nursing, and working out.

How about a new store? You could call it Victoria's Reality. It would sell plush thick bathrobes, instead of those cold, silk ones. They'd carry sturdy underwire bras with matching underwear. Forgo the lace and give us underwear that has some stretch to it and goes up at least past our hip bones.

At a certain point, I traded sexy for comfort. I think a good day is when I wear a matching bra and underwear. And trust me, when you wear that your husband will notice.

IT'S ALL IN THE JEANS

Just because we're moms doesn't mean we don't want to look good. So yes. I am all about comfort, but I didn't want to wear anything that could fall into the category of, well, mom pants.

The last time I bought jeans, they were skinny jeans. Those should come with a sticker that reads, “These jeans are skinny, whereas you might not be.” It’s the worst fashion concept of the last decade. For the past six months, I am only comfortable wearing skinny jeans if I can wear something long and oversized with them. A football jersey is perfect.

So in my quest to find the perfect pair of non-mom pants, I spent an hour looking for jeans. I even tried to take budget out of it and just get what I really like. First there were the ones that have the mock rips in them. I just can’t bring myself to pay for something torn. I can easily rip the clothes I have now for free.

Then there are the ones that are bedazzled. On the pockets they have blingy decorations on them. Those designs are like a magnet for people’s eyes. And my back end really doesn’t need that kind of attention.

Of course there were more skinny jeans. Nope. Been there, done that.

The boot cut jeans were a possibility. But I always feel that I actually have to wear boots whenever I wear the jeans. I feel like a traitor wearing itsy bitsy ankle shoes with them. It’s just not right.

I finally found something I liked. They were Gloria Vanderbilt. Her son is Anderson Cooper, and who doesn't love him, right? Okay, so that brand hasn't really been big since the 1980s, but the sticky tag on the front read "LOOK SLIMMER." Now we're talking. I mean they didn't say you'll look skinny, but simply slimmer. That sounds realistic. It's like a nice way of saying you won't look great, but you won't look so bad either.

Once I got home with my new jeans, my older son wanted to see what I bought. I excitedly showed him the jeans and asked what he thought.

"They look like hip hop jeans. Like you would wear those and be looking for a hip hop guy."

I figured at best, I'd snag a guy from the Village People.

Whatever. Hip hop jeans have got to be a step up from mom pants, right?

DO I LOOK LIKE A MOM IN THIS DRESS?

I remember before I had kids I would see women 10 years after high school or college. I used to wonder what happened to them. They looked, well, different. It was as if their hair wasn't kept up, and they put on weight. They looked tired. How naive.

I get it now. Part of it is age. But after you have kids, a lot of things change. We look like (gasp) moms!

That's why when I go shopping or go to the salon, I feel more polished. The problem is now it all has to be mapped out. What's the budget? What style and color do I want? What stores do I want to go to and when do they open? Add kids to that map, and it's a three-ring circus. I'm certain of this as I have tried.

We recently had a wedding to attend, so I stopped at the area's largest shoe warehouse to find shoes. Seriously, they gotta have 3,000 pair of shoes. My thought has been if you go there and can't find shoes, you either A) really didn't look, or B) your feet are a size 15. In my case, it was option C) because I had my kids with me. Their behavior was fine, but they were running up to me with every shoe they thought I would like. As you might imagine, this took a while.

My kids meant well, and they tried to be helpful.

"Mom, try this."

A stiletto? So not gonna happen.

"Can you try this one?" They would ask excitedly.

"No. That's a size 6. Mommy is a 10."

Mysteriously, since childbirth my left foot is an 11. For me, shoe shopping is like finding a two-piece bathing suit. The same size rarely fits both parts.

"No. Not that one either. It's the wrong color."

I knew that finding a dress would prove to be even worse than my recent jean and shoe shopping adventures, so I decided to spare the boys (and my sanity) and go alone. My style has become predictable, and I wanted to try something different. I kept second guessing myself and thinking, *Do I look like a mom in this?*

The dressing room was filled with girls half my age. It was such a change from hanging with the boys. Some of the girls were chatting and complimenting each other. They were discussing their weekend plans. Then one of them said, "No way! This looked much different on the hanger. It doesn't look good on me. It's more for like an older Cougar type." Oooh. Cougar wear? I was tempted to ask her to bring down my way.

After I got home with a couple dresses I bought, I decided to put on a mini fashion show for the family. I wasn't thinking my husband and boys were going to jump for joy, but I was hoping to get a positive response. Hoping was a mistake.

My youngest pointed to my stomach area and noted, "It looks like there is a baby in there."

"Yeah I can see some of your tummy, Mom."

I learned two things: **1)** Family approval of ones wardrobe is overrated. **2)** Sweat pants and an oversized t-shirt can serve you well for a long time.

THE LADIES ROOM

I never thought one could find quiet and comfort in the bathroom. And I was right. But you can't fault me for trying.

You'll find an entry in this book about our one-holer house. That means there is one toilet. For all of us. My advice? If your kids are in diapers when you are looking at homes to buy, don't forget that at some point the goal is to potty train them. Buy a house with more than one toilet. Even if the second bathroom is scary and covered in cobwebs in the basement. Or get a really big ice cream pail.

I don't want to give the impression that I go into the bathroom and sprawl out on the floor to relax. First of all, it's too small. It's like 5' by 5'. Secondly, I live with males, and they tend to miss the toilet. Maybe it's just me, but lying on the bathroom floor and smelling urine doesn't seem like a great way to relax.

But sometimes it's nice to do your duty and not be rushed. You know, let nature take its time. Just doesn't work that way. It appears that some type of alarm goes off whenever I close the door to the bathroom. I'm pretty sure it says, "MOM IS IN THE BATHROOM. EVEN IF YOU JUST USED THE BATHROOM OR HELD IT FOR THE PAST 30 MINUTES, YOU SHOULD NOW ENTER THE BATROOM. REPEAT. MOM IS IN THE BATHROOM."

Don't you love taking baths? People say it is a good way to relax. Not so much in the one-holer house. There seems to be a lure to the bathroom when I do take a bath. I get that the boys need to use the toilet. But it would be preferable if they could get in and get out. I think they talk more through that shower curtain to each other than they do any other time. Then just as they finish their task, they like to poke their head around the curtain. That's when it officially takes a creepy turn.

Eventually, they leave me in peace and serenity. With a tub full of water that's now cold. With the smell of poop looming in the air. We really need to get a lock on that door soon. Or buy a two-holer house.

DON'T EVEN TRY TO DO IT ALL

One reason we moms get easily stressed is the fantasy that we can have it all—a husband, career, kids, and a social life.

Before I had it all, I remember thinking, *How hard could it be? I'll have a house, a husband, a very grown-up job, and kids*. Now I realize that would all be easy if the house were self-cleaning. And if the husband didn't have to put in so many hours at work. And if the kids never got colds. And if the grass was always that perfect shade of green. And if someone would kindly do all the grocery shopping. And the cooking. And if the stocks we bought were actually worth something.

Sure. We can have it all. You bet. But it's like a smorgasbord. It's all there for you to choose from. Fancy cheeses, filet mignon, mashed potatoes, green beans, pork 'n beans, those weanie things on toothpicks, bacon-wrapped chestnuts, carrots, broccoli (pass), salmon, sweet corn, corn on the cob, bread, gobs of butter. Even dessert. It's all there. You can eat it all. Go ahead eat it. Yeah. How are you feeling now? It's like a real life Alka-Seltzer commercial. You take too much, and you will combust.

It's not far from how it is with life. Sometimes there's just too much going on. But we feel compelled to do it all. Why? Maybe it's just our nature. Frankly, the older I get I feel that perfection is overrated. Maybe I'm just getting lazy. Or tired. Or realistic.

Recently, a friend of mine found out she mailed a card that was supposed to have a check in it. She accidentally forgot to put the check in before mailing the card. In an email to me, she asked, "Can you tell that I'm coming unglued?"

I was actually relieved to read that email.

I'm not the only one, I thought.

One day, I threw a check away. Yes. In the garbage. It took me less than 10 seconds to grab the check from the pile of mail. Then it took me more than 10 minutes searching through the garbage can for it. I was busy going through the mail and listening to voice messages and thinking about making dinner and just absent mindedly threw the check in the garbage.

Another friend who has five children and is married

told me she needs a couple hours a week just to think. She said she needs to go somewhere like Dunkin' Donuts just to gather her thoughts. I was thinking somewhere *not* to have to think sounded like a good place. And, yeah, if donuts are served, even better!

As women, we tend to think it's all gotta get done, and we have to be the ones to do it. But if we are always doing it, no one else has the chance to. So, yeah. We can have it all. And maybe even at one time. But just a heads-up: Something will likely end up in the garbage.

IT TAKES A VILLAGE

I'm not a huge fan of clichés, campaigns, or slogans because it seems that people hide behind them. But there is an African proverb, "It takes a village to raise a child." The more I parent, the more I see that that is so true. You can't do it alone.

When you're pregnant, everybody wants to give you advice. The problem is, you might not be ready for it. I wanted to go through things without having people tell me how it was gonna go. SPOLER ALERT: Labor is intense. Thanks for the heads-up.

But at some point, you might want to rely on others—for you and for your children's sake. I call it sharing the gift of mom. Like the friend who asked if my kids would like to come spend the day at her house because they were off school. That was a big gift.

Normally when the kids have off, it makes my skin tighten up. Not the kind of skin tightening that takes the crow's feet away. The kind that just adds another layer of physical stress. The kind that's a direct result of trying to figure out child care for the kids when there's no school.

My friend makes it seem effortless. After making banana bread, she took the kids to a museum, out for lunch, and to a movie. For me, just the thought of all that is a lot of work. Each time I arrive to pick up my kids from her house, they frown and tell me they don't want to leave.

So, yeah. We all have gifts. One of the nicest things you can do with the gift of being a good mom is share yourself with other moms. And your banana bread.

ME? A SOCCER MOM?

It sure is interesting how things change once you have kids. Including your attitude.

I really used to despise two things on cars: the signs that said "Baby On Board" and the stickers that said, "Soccer Mom." I'm not sure why I had such distaste for those things. The only thing I can think of is that I couldn't relate. I wasn't part of the club. Yet.

I am not proud of this story, but it's part of my history and again my attitude was different before kids entered the picture.

I was in line at the bank drive-thru, vying for the next open teller. Next to me was a minivan. A minivan with kids in it. A minivan with kids and that sticker. Soccer mom. I was neck and neck with a soccer mom. I knew my Mercedes sedan could smoke her minivan any day.

When it was go-time, I got the open spot before her. I remember the look on her face of shock as she laid on her horn. My response? "Nice way to act, soccer mom! With your kids in the car!"

Shameful behavior on my part. But I've grown much since then. I now would think to let someone with small kids go before me. She might have had a crying screaming baby in the car. Her minivan is probably an extension of her office. She was working and trying to do her job just like the rest of us.

Ironically, I am now a soccer mom. Only I don't have the sticker in the window of my SUV. Yet.

THERE'S A BUMPER STICKER FOR THAT

If soccer isn't your thing, no worries. You have a plethora of bumper stickers from which to choose.

How about the Irish Dancers? Their bumper stickers are a bit more colorful than the soccer mom stickers. I'm not Irish, but I would consider joining just for the wigs! Perfect ringlets every time!

Or maybe you want to join the gymnast moms. I need to warn you though. These are not for the moms who are slackers. The better your kid gets at gymnastics, the higher level they advance. The higher the level, the more often they have to be at the gym. The more often they are at the gym, the more it's gonna cost you. So if you have like two to four spare nights a week and an extra $75 to $200 a week, this might be the group for you. We tried it for a while, but at certain point, our son just sat on the mat, rolling around and not at all interested in taking part in the routines. I realized that he could roll around on the floor at home. For free.

When your kids are school-age, make way for the PTO moms. Word to the wise: If you're a mom who doesn't want to do much extra, this is so not the group for you. These ladies know how to get stuff done. They have the ability to organize an auction, picnic, teacher appreciation day, secret Santa shop, root beer float day, school dance, and anything else that might bring the school camaraderie, funds, and notoriety.

The stay-at-home moms are a close-knit group. To give you a heads-up on this group, do not ever say, "Oh, so you don't work." Ever. I tried being a stay-at-home mom for the first few years of having kids. One word: overwhelming.

When you stay at home, some people don't get it. They assume you're having crumpets and tea. What with all that time you have, you know, just staying at home. Biggest. Misconception. Ever! Puke, laundry, doctor appointments, play dates, grocery shopping, car maintenance, lawn care, UPS drop offs. All of that gets done with a kid in tow! Breastfeeding while in the lobby of the Firestone dealer is your reality.

When you stay at home with your kids, your home is your office. When you stay home, you are constantly using things, so your house is hard to keep clean. The diapers, the laundry, the kitchen floor. It's a cleaning cycle that feels like it will never end.

If you stay at home, you're responsible for feeding yourself and your kids. Your home provides the cafeteria. Hence this will lead back to the laundry and the kitchen floor.

Moms who stay at home don't get sick days. Nope. There's no number to call in sick to! I recall being sick with a newborn and a toddler. I was sure my husband would not go to work that morning. Wishful thinking! I stared at the door as he left, bawling. How was I going to take care of these kids when I could barely move?

As I was wasting what energy I did have crying, my friend called. She just happened to call on her way to work.

I know she was freaked out when I answered the phone crying. She told me she would go in to her job that day but then call in and help me the next day. Just hearing that brought relief.

Which leads to the reality that staying at home can lead to feeling isolated. You don't get to hang out around the water cooler and chat it up with your co-workers at 9 in the morning. No. By 9 am, you're standing next to a Diaper Genie and changing your kid's outfit—for the second time that morning. You don't buy cool new outfits to wear to the office. You buy stuff made of cotton that does not require ironing and cleans up well. You trade in a briefcase for a diaper bag.

When you stay at home, you don't get bonuses, raises, or a plaque that says you're the employee of the month. When you stay at home, you aren't even sure you're doing a good job. No one tells you!

When staying at home has taken its toll on you, you'll know. When you freak out when you notice that the schedule from 6 am until noon on PBS has changed, it might be time. When you cry just looking at your crisp white business shirts, it might be time. When your diet consists of animal crackers and juice boxes, it might be time. When you know every McDonald's within a 20-mile radius with the play equipment, it might be time. When you engage the mail carrier in conversation, it may be time.

MOM, FOR HIRE

At some point, you might decide that maybe working outside the home is better for you and your family. That comes with its own set of circumstances.

The idea of leaving my kids with other people for the bulk of the day was horrifying. What if they cry all day? What if the workers don't understand their needs?

They first day I began working out of the house, I felt sick. Miles was three years old at the time, and when I dropped him off, he was totally at home. Max not so much. He wailed as I walked away. My heart sank. What kind of mother was I?

For three weeks, Max would cry when I left him. For three weeks, I would stand outside the room he was in and wait until he stopped crying. Usually it was only 60 seconds. But they were painfully long 60 seconds.

I resented that I had to work outside the home, but I knew the kids were fine. Thriving actually. I was back in the world of dry-clean-only clothes. Water cooler chit chat. Adult lunches!

But even when you think it's what is best for you, you still wonder. For me, it's when I'm driving to work and I see a group of moms pushing strollers and drinking Starbucks coffee. The grass is always greener. But, man, that Starbucks looks good.

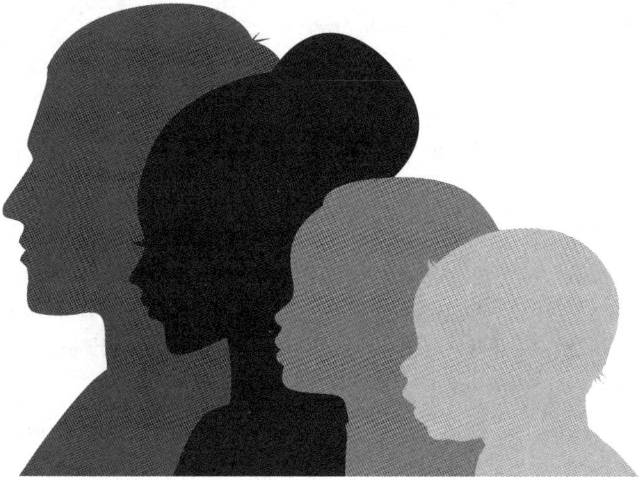

8

Things I Think About

WHAT IS GOD LIKE?

For many people who believe in God, there's a visual that goes along with it. The idea of believing in someone or something might seem incomplete without a look to go along with it. Yep. Even God has a profile picture. Often it's a fluffy image, barely there. Somewhere between the Pillsbury Doughboy and the Michelin Man, with a toga style outfit.

Kids try to figure God out as well. Who didn't think God was angry when we heard the constant thunder during a bad storm? My son Max told me when God gets upset he makes tornadoes happen. He also heard that if you give God the finger, he'll give you the finger right back! You show 'em, God!

But then imagine having this idea of what God looks like all to have that change. It happened at our house.

Our kids get a kick out of music videos. They love to do their little dances complete with costume changes.

One afternoon, a music video featuring James Brown came on. My husband got excited and announced, "It's the godfather of soul!"

My youngest son was even more excited. "That's God the Father? That's what he looks like?"

It took a few minutes, but we were finally able to explain the difference between the God the Father and the godfather of soul. But then, really, who knows? Maybe they are the same person.

DO YOU REALLY NEED TO KNOW THAT?

The curiosity of children is amazing. From rocks to dragons, from the planets to the ocean. They just have an insatiable appetite to lean more. At some point, they're going to want to know where babies came from.

At six and seven, my boys thought they had it figured out. They pretty much believed that a mommy would eat a lot of food. Then when her belly got too full, the baby would come out. "A" for effort. The eating a lot and big belly was right on from my experience.

But by ages seven and eight, my sons were modifying that theory. My older son is a huge science buff, and he had heard about DNA. But he couldn't figure out how Daddy's DNA mixed with mine.

When my sons were eight and nine, I caved. I couldn't have them believing in a stork or baby fairy. I gave them the low-down-dirty details on where babies really came from. Okay, actually I told them that moms and dads put their private parts together, which makes a baby. My youngest went to his bedroom upon hearing that, but my oldest just sat there with a look of horror on his face. I realized that there was no turning back, but I also realized I might have damaged him for life.

Finally, when he did speak, he asked, "Why would you do that?"

I thought, *Quick, think of something*. I can still see his sad and confused eyes looking at me.

And then I did it. I threw my husband under the bus. I told my son it was his father's idea. Suddenly, the stork story didn't seem so bad.

BELIEVE IT OR NOT

Childhood is supposed to include innocence, naiveté, and even a little magic. Enter the Tooth Fairy, the Easter Bunny, and Santa. They're all a big part of many kids' lives. But sometimes to keep the whole charade going, you feel like a liar.

Think about it. We tell our kids they're safe in our home. We have sturdy doors with strong locks. We install security systems. Yep. We're all safe, and no one can get in the house. Except the Tooth Fairy, the Easter Bunny, and Santa. It sounds kinda hypocritical.

You have to be on top of your game when it comes to these characters. Miles once asked me, "Does the Tooth Fairy have wings?" I said yes because I thought she was somehow related to Peter Pan.

Santa does watch you. And has a very strict budget. (I know firsthand this one is really not a lie.) Oh, and he's cousins with St. Nick. I think. And they hang with Kris Kringle. You get yourself in deeper and deeper with each detail.

At school, they talk about the Blanket Fairy. I'm guessing that's the one that takes away your baby blanket when you no longer need it. I'm waiting to be asked were they take all of those blankets after they retrieve them.

I'd be remiss if I didn't mention the Easter Bunny. This one baffles me the most. See, the bunnies in our backyard are small and hop around on four legs. They don't wear clothes. But the ones at the mall are like six and a half feet tall and standing on two legs. Honestly, they're kind of creepy. Sort of what you would expect to see in a sci-fi film. And they're always sporting very snappy outfits. And why are they hiding eggs? They don't even lay eggs. I propose we have an Easter Chicken.

The last time Miles lost a tooth, I was in his room right after he'd found money from the Tooth Fairy. He looked up at me and asked, "Mom, did Dad put the money under my pillow?"

I thought, *Now is the time. Explain to him that the Tooth Fairy isn't real*. But as soon as I had that thought, I felt sad.

I told him he could ask his dad to find out. He just smiled and replied, "No. I'm pretty sure the Tooth Fairy is real." Whew.

There's something almost sacred about that childhood magic. These beliefs bring so much happiness to kids. How dare I bring an end to that? Besides, there are braces on the horizon, and the Tooth Fairy will most certainly be contributing to that.

THE QUESTIONS I'M CLUELESS ABOUT

I encourage my boys to ask questions. That's a great way to learn. The problem is I can't answer many of their questions. Every day it becomes apparent that I'm really not smart. Honestly, I'm fine with that. I just don't want them to find out. Because if they find out, then others are sure to follow. What if kids tease then on the playground, chanting, "Your Mommy's not smart! Your Mommy's not smart!"

So I have decided to at least appear to know some things. Whenever possible, I give an answer that sounds good.

What is the highest number?

Gazillion.

How do snakes hear?

Snakes are dangerous, and we need to worry more about hearing *them*.

How hot is the sun?

Super hot.

When is kid's day?

Seriously? Every day.

Is Kris Kringle related to Santa Clause?

Yes. But they don't hang out much because they have so much work to do.

Will my penis grow when I'm adult?

I hope so.

Can a cheetah run faster than a car?

Let's hope not. You don't see a cheetah now do you?

How does Santa know if we're in a different town for Christmas?

Mommy and Santa are close. Very close.

Do babies come out of your butt?

No, but it feels like it.

Why don't we walk around naked?

Because many of our bodies don't look so good as we get older. You'll grow to appreciate certain parts being covered up.

If I was born in the year of the tiger, would I be 13?

Maybe. But you were born in 2004.

Why do bunnies eat their poop?

Umm, do they really do that? Maybe they think they're chocolate chips. And no, you may not have bunny for a pet.

Why do we have hair on our legs?

So men look manly and women can spend 15 minutes a week shaving it off.

Why was Earth created?

So we'd have somewhere to live.

How do big glaciers stay afloat?

Life jackets?

How many rings does Saturn have?

Wait. Do you mean the car or the planet?

Do you know about Corvettes, Mustangs, and Camaros?

Yes. They are expensive and hard to get car seats in.

And when all else fails and I am at the height of clueless-ness, I usually say, **"Ask your Dad."**

YOU'RE NOT REALLY GONNA BE SICK, ARE YOU?

Somehow whenever the kids get sick, it's never convenient. As a parent, it can feel like your whole world is thrown off when your child is ill.

One particular morning, my son Max was coughing so much that we thought maybe he should stay home. We asked if he wanted to go to daycare, and he said yes. I'm not sure why we decided it was his decision to stay home or go to daycare. Maybe we thought maybe the cough would calm down as the morning wears on. Or not.

On our drive to daycare, I convinced him to take cough

drop. I did that whole "Mmmm, it's really good. Tastes like candy" thing. The thing that your pediatrician tells you not to do. Yeah, I did that.

Well that trick is old news and didn't work.

"It's gonna be spicy," he said and reluctantly took it.

I peered at him through the rearview mirror and see him grimacing.

"You don't like the cough drop do you?" I asked. "Uh uh."

I leaned over to the glove box to find a napkin (thank you, McDonald's) and reached back to give it to him to spit into. Then he said in a sad little voice, "I think I'm gonna throw up."

Oh, man. I looked around for things to give him in lieu of a toilet. Wet wipes and McDonald's straws wouldn't do the job. Nothing brings out the Starsky and Hutch in you like a kid who says he's gonna be sick.

"Okay, honey, let Mommy pull over."

I stepped on the gas and merged right, hoping not to upset the long line of fellow morning commuters. I didn't have time for rude hand gestures and comments about bad lady drivers. That would have been a great time for one of those cool flashing lights for the top of the car.

The threat of vomit is a great motivator. It took me just under 30 seconds to find a park to pull over at. I quickly jumped out the driver side and met him at his door.

Just in time. Each time he heaved, I tried not to gag myself, while hearing my older son groan and say, "Oh gross!" Of course, he just had to look.

So I am trying to not puke, keep my little guy calm, and listen to how disgusted my other son is.

At one point, I was going back and forth, saying, "It's okay honey. You're gonna be alright" to one kid, and "Will you please shut up!" to the other one adding his commentary. The little guy was still getting sick, and then the older one started crying. "Mom, please don't tell me to shut up!"

To top it off, we were in a neighboring suburb, and I was worried the cops were going to come and start asking questions. I was pretty sure the stench of vomit would give me a free pass.

THEY WILL ASSUME YOU CAN DO ANYTHING

For a while, it seems that as a parent you can do no wrong. When your babies need something, you make it magically appear. When they get tired, you make sure they get a nap. You even have a snack for them when they wake up.

When they scrape their knees, your kisses ease the pain. When they're frightened, a hug from you calms them down. You get the medicine in and the bugs out.

But at a certain point, the requests get pretty big. A couple years ago Max asked for a little sister. And Miles had to put in his order as well. He wanted twins! When we moms are good, we're good, but there are some things we just can't do.

DAD'S MORE...EVERYTHING

For the first few years, it seems like we moms are the favored parent. Perhaps it's because we housed them for almost 10 months. Yeah, and breastfeeding definitely pulls them our way. But then things slowly taper off. My sister-in-law once said that by the time boys are four or five, you're toast.

So maybe not quite toast. More like a bagel. The half of bagel at the bottom of the bag. Everyone likes it, but they're just tired of the flavor. So they sort of ignore it, thinking one day they'll go back to it.

I have been told countless times by my kids that my husband is more fun. Maybe that makes for a good balance because I'm more of a worrier. For example, when he takes the boys fishing, I obsess on one of them getting a hook caught on the other one. If they go sledding, I wonder if they're too cold. While they are out shopping, I keep looking at the time, knowing bedtime is approaching. On road trips, I wonder if everyone has their seatbelts buckled. Yeah. I pretty much suck the life out of the party. Dad's more fun.

And then there's this. My boys have said, "Not to be mean, but I think Dad paid more attention in school, because he's a little smarter than you." So much for the "Smart Mom Award."

But what about all the stuff that Dad can't do? Like paint his nails while talking on the phone? Or putting on panty hose without ripping them. Or remembering play dates, birthday parties, and dance lessons. Where's the credit for that?

On the other hand, if Dad is really smarter, then all questions should be directed to him. Therefore giving me more time to chat with friends, head to Target, and grab a latte from Starbucks. Maybe being smart is overrated.

Naturally, you realize that you and your husband do things differently, but in case you misplace that realization, your kids will be happy to point it out to you on more than one occasion. The words are the same each time. "Dad doesn't do it like that." Each time it may be tempting to tell them that dad does it wrong. But that wouldn't be nice. And probably not even true.

If you've ever made instant oatmeal, you know that the directions are three steps. Still, my husband and I do it differently. He pours the boiling milk into the oatmeal; I boil the milk with the oatmeal in the bowl.

He folds their shirts in thirds. I fold them in half. He likes them to take up less room, and I want them to look like they do on the shelves at the Gap.

Kids need to be able to adapt. It's fine that mom and dad do things differently. Well, except that toilet paper thing. The paper has to go under.

PINK VS. BLUE

Are girls and boys really that different? I'm not a psychologist. If I were, I would be writing some incredibly intellectual piece on why kids do what they do. That's not me. I write what I see my kids do. Just like when I decided to not just give them the stereotypical "boy toys." I gave them a doll. They immediately ripped her dress off and dragged her along the floor. That was the last doll they played with.

As much as I want to believe that it's how we nurture our kids, there must be a whole lot of nature in there as well. I sit in awe watching girls play together. They giggle and smile sweetly, sitting relatively still, busy with their coloring books. My older son just showed me a spot on the basement wall where he drew his name.

You get what you get. That might be the best way to look at it. Kind of like those grab bags you can buy at flea markets and rummage sales. The difference is you can re-gift what's in the bags if you don't like it. That's not so cool to do with kids.

THAT MOM ISN'T YOU, AND THAT'S OKAY

I used to be a perfectionist. Or tried to be. But honestly, being a perfectionist is hard work, and well, that's not fun. I wouldn't say I'm a sloth, but my standards of needing to do a good job have changed. I don't know if it's age, low energy, or laziness, but my standards are not the same as they used to be. Some moms can do things really well. I admire them. However, it kinda sets the bar high for us low achievers.

One woman ran the Chicago marathon and gave birth afterward—as in the same day! She ran half and walked the other half. I walked like 15 minutes a few times a week for the first trimester with my oldest son. Then I convinced myself why bother. I was big as a house anyway, and I treated myself to chili cheese dogs a few times a week.

There's more. When her contractions became regular, she stopped for a bite to eat before going to the hospital! I was at the hospital when the contractions weren't regular. *Please, please don't send me home. I like it here. You have cable TV, room service, and a bed that reclines!*

This year, I was excited to bring a treat to school for my son's birthday. I met with his teachers to find out if that was okay and how much I should bring. One teacher almost drooled as she recalled how another mom brought in chocolate covered bananas to share for her child's birthday. I can only imagine how disappointed she was with my store-bought donut holes. But I bought three different flavors. That has to count for something.

The moms who look flawless really amaze me. Makeup done. Hair done. Stylish outfits. It seems that when I have that entire combo going, someone seems surprised and can't resist asking what the special occasion is. Generally, it's because I actually picked out the outfit the night before, had just been to the salon, and had time to put makeup on my whole face, not just eyeliner and blush.

Truthfully, I admire people who can do things and do them well. Moms need to support other moms because we each bring something to the table. Having said that, I wonder if it works both ways. What's the likelihood one of them is in awe looking at me trying to figure out, How does she pull off that bed head hair look so well?

IT'S NOT JUST YOU

Misery loves company. We've all heard that saying more than a few times. There's probably a lot of truth to that, but the word misery just sounds so-miserable. So maybe we can put a new twist to an old cliché? Like, Moms love company.

We tend to be so focused on our own kids. Perhaps too focused. We zero in on their words, their grades, their behaviors. I recall being so upset when in K5 my son got in trouble for yelling in class. A note in his backpack said, "I yelled 'butt' in class."

After I had chastised my son for 10 minutes, he asked me if I had seen the other side of the note. It read, "I yelled 'penis' in class." My first thought was to write back to his teacher and say "Don't send any more notes home until he says 'vagina.'" After more consideration, I realized that would not foster a very good relationship with his teacher.

But when I first saw the note I was mortified. I kept thinking, *Why would he say these things? I never go around saying "penis."* What have I done wrong? And then my son told me that other kids were saying the same things. They would all say the words and then giggle. I was so happy when he told me that. I almost didn't care anymore what words he had said.

Of course, our kids aren't the only ones doing the things they do. But when their behavior is on the negative side, it tends to feel that way. In the end, maybe it does come down to the fact that we do love company. There's a certain amount of comfort in knowing it's not just us. Like realizing other moms are struggling to lose weight. Or finding out other women are trying to balance work, kids, and marriage. No one ever wants to be the odd one out.

As you journey through parenthood, keep in mind that all of us have something going on when it comes to our children. Likely a lot of somethings. So if your kid says a naughty word in class, just know there are a million other moms going through something similar. Yep, millions of kids blurting out "butt" in class every day. You're in good company.

THE KIDS GET IT

Do we talk enough? Never mind if your husband tells you too much. But I mean as women, as parents, are we taking the time to just have a chat with each other? Having kids gives us an instant connection.

Kids get it. Watch them. Listen to them. They take the time. As we're telling them it's time to get in the car, they're chatting it up with the neighbors, the mail carrier, people passing by, and stray animals.

And what better place to chat it up than the grocery store. Aisle 3 specifically. The one we found with a little girl unable to decide which Lunchable she should get. Her father stood back, clearly not well versed in this area.

My son Miles reached over her head, pulled one down, and explained to her, "This kind is bigger, and you get more food."

She smiled at her dad, who looked at me and asked, "Are the pizza ones any good?"

Before I could answer, Max piped in. "Yeah. Those are good too if you like pizza."

So for the next three minutes, my boys and the adorable girl in sparkly shoes discussed their options of prepackaged food. Ham and cheese? Nachos? Turkey and cheese?

It wasn't a concern that one of them liked to wear dresses and the others blew out the knees of his jeans. They found common ground.

That same day, we went to a park to burn off some energy and met some boys who were very excited to show off their new bikes. And they weren't the only ones. There was another boy with a new mountain bike, a little guy with training wheels, and one on a trike. It was like the United Nations of all things with wheels.

It didn't matter that they were different ages and sizes. At first they all crept closer and closer together without a word, and then Miles asked the group, "Wanna race?"

It was on! You could almost see a trail of testosterone behind them. The boys were making car sounds, pedaling as fast as they could, and then slamming on the brakes to make skid marks.

Adult conversation should be that easy too. So maybe next time you pull up to a stoplight and notice another mom in a minivan next to you, you could rev up you engine, roll down your window, and ask her if she wants to race. Okay, maybe not. But how about asking another mom is she wants to share a Lunchable with you? I suggest the super big ones; they come with a juice box and chocolate.

FROM A CHILD'S VIEW

It's so easy to get stressed out about life. The grown-up world is quite a serious place to be. But it wasn't always that way. Once upon a time we too were kids.

Tonight Max is going to his first sleepover. He has been talking about it for three weeks, ever since his friend mentioned it. He hit a new level of excitement when he got the invitation in the mail. He said he and his friends were going to stay up late and play games. When was the last time you got that excited to see your friends—four days in advance?

We recently visited one of my brothers and sister-in-law. The boys were happy to take a trip, but what did they get more juiced up about? A rope swing in the yard. And a pick ax. Does that sound like something you'd write home about?

When there are functions at school in the evening, they beg to go. But for most of us, once we clock out at 5:00 pm, it's sayonara!

We grumble in the airport waiting for a connecting

flight. The kids are squealing with delight that there is another horizontal escalator.

Max almost stopped in his tracks when he saw our coffee maker on the counter. "What's that?" he asked.

We rarely use it so I had to explain to him that it was a coffee maker and that instead of going to Starbucks I could make coffee at home. The blank stare on his face told me he still didn't understand. Or maybe he was disappointed because no Starbucks meant no over-sized cookie for him.

The next morning, the distinct, sweet smell of hazelnut lured him from his room to the kitchen. Max couldn't contain his excitement. "Dad, look it's dripping down. It's making the coffee!"

He ran to the top of the stairs to let his brother in on this new found piece of technology. He was so flustered he could barely talk. So instead he gave him the hand signal that means, "Come quick. You gotta see this!"

And there they were, side by side, admiring the coffee maker in all her glory. One drip after another.

They have a Wii. They've been on a plane. They went to the Grand Canyon. But still, this simple appliance gave them a thrill. Just wait 'til we get a dishwasher.

Okay, so maybe a pick ax won't do it for you. But when you feel like you're overwhelmed, remember that at one time it really was the simple things that made you smile. And maybe just thinking about that will get you through the rough spots.

TALK TO YOUR YOUNGER SELF

As you think back to your youth, do you marvel at all the ridiculous things you did? Wearing ill-fitting shoes because they were cute. Or dating a guy who you knew was not good for you. Maybe you skipped a whole week of class in college but you rarely missed happy hour.

It's interesting how as time goes on our past seems to be filled with bad decisions, guilt, and regret. Admittedly, we often had a lot of fun before we came to that realization. But maybe we can avoid that looking back with disappointment feeling.

If you think about it, it's likely that in 10 or 20 years, you'll look back at these child-rearing years and think, If only I had...

Obviously, mistakes will be made. But we might be able to minimize those by thinking ahead. (I know. Who has time for that right?) But it couldn't hurt to try.

Here's a list to start with:

Stop worrying. It'll stress you out. Then you'll get sick and worry about that!

Make the most of being pregnant. It might be the only time that total stranger's open doors, let you cut in line, and give you a smile for no reason.

Let the baby cry to sleep. It's either you or him.

Don't forget your husband. When the kids leave for college, he'll still be there.

Stop comparing yourself to other moms. They have problems too. Maybe even more than you.

Don't feel guilty if you're doing what is best for your children. You can give them guilt trips later by reminding them how much you sacrificed for them.

Don't try to believe you can have it all at once. You might be able to, but you'll be a zombie, your house will be a total mess, and your kids and husband will be miserable.

Take care of yourself. Don't see it as selfish, but rather self-preservation.

Let the house be messy. As long as there is glitter, glue, animal crackers, runny noses, rain, dirt, orange juice, crayons, cereal, Halloween candy, pets, poop, raisins, Hot Wheels, Barbie Dolls, DVDs, toothpaste, shoes, and toilets, it's gonna get messy.

Don't worry about what you forgot to pick up at the grocery store. There's a good chance you'll be back there tomorrow.

Try not to get too worked up about labor. Look at how many people there are in the world. It can't be that bad.

Try to see the humorous side to things. If you laugh hard enough, you'll wet your pants. Now that's funny.

It's okay not to have the last word. Just think it.

Find a place to have a few moments alone when you need it. Other than the bathroom or Starbucks.

Apologize to your kids when you screw up. They may take pity on you and visit you when you're old.

Show affection to your spouse or partner. Your kids won't get those social cues from reality TV, the playground, or their electronic gadgets.

Ask for help. You'll need it.

Mistakes will be made. Don't beat yourself over them. Your kids will handle that for you.

GET YOUR LAUGH ON

Did you laugh a lot as a kid? So much that the teacher would scold you? The kind of laugh that would get you a stern look from your parents if it happened in church?

When is the last time you really laughed? I'm not talking about the fake laugh you make when your husband's boss cracks a joke. I'm talking about the real unadulterated laugh-until-you-pee-in-your-pants laugh. You might not even recall the last time you laughed like that. Maybe you have a friend that gets you going. My friend Jody does that for me. It's like a secret language we speak, and we just giggle like kids.

Movies, humor books, old photo albums, and comedy shows are just a few ideas of ways to get laughing. And it feels so good. It's almost better than sex. But don't tell your husband that.

There are a lot of tears with pregnancy, childbirth, and parenting. But we can only cry so much. Watch kids. They laugh constantly. At almost anything. Go on: Find your inner funny and pee your pants!

BE GRATEFUL

Often, life as a parent can get to a point that seems unbearable. Sometimes you have to really step back and look at what you have so you don't just walk out the door—forever.

As I'm rushing to drive my boys to school, I see groups of moms, pushing strollers and walking their young kids to school. In the cup holder, I see cups with the insignia of a popular coffee chain. They drop their kids off at school and head back home. To me they look refreshed and carefree.

Meanwhile, my guys are in the backseat fighting over the armrest and whose backpack is encroaching on the other's designated territory. My threats to pull the car over are ignored, and the chaos in the backseat continues.

But then I think back to the period of time where I was home during the day with the boys. Sure I had a stroller, but I resented it because over time it became much like that lawn chair from Charlie Brown. The one that kept collapsing. And I also stopped at the popular coffee shop. I drank so much coffee I was wide awake at midnight.

And when you are at home with the kids, well, you don't get a lot of adult stimulation. By 9 in the morning I'd had it with television. Thomas the Trains' accent got old real quick. And quite frankly the Teletubbies were a bit creepy. They were like a cross between the Pillsbury Doughboy and some type of alien. And they talked more baby gibberish than a real baby!

Most nights, my husband puts the boys to bed. It's their ritual. He meets them at the bottom of the staircase and races them upstairs. Sometimes he wins, and sometimes they beat him. Then instead of brushing their teeth the three of them are rolling around and wrestling. My initial response is to raise my voice and tell the kids that I'm going to tell their dentist they aren't brushing teeth and that their teeth will rot. But lately, I try to hear the familiar thumps on the ceiling as a sign of how blessed we are.

I have husband who enjoys being a dad. And I have two healthy kids who adore him. And that feeling lasts for a while. And then-someone breaks something. Yep. The party is over.

We think the grass is greener. No it's not. It's a different shade. And who wants perfect green grass? Do you know how much work that is? It's the same with kids. No I don't mean that they are different shades of green. Rather, they come with different talents, challenges, strengths, and weaknesses.

My boys have an amazing amount of energy. They're always moving. Why I'm not a size four because of running after them is a mystery to me. I don't mean they're mischievous. They go for seven-mile bike rides with my husband, skateboard for two hours at a time, kick around the soccer ball until it's tattered.

A friend of mine said to me that it's easier to calm a spirited child than add energy to a laid-back child. That made so much sense. It might take us awhile, but there's something to be said about embracing our kids—everything about them.

You'll come to see that what you think are problems are merely just inconveniences. I think about parents who are at a hospital knowing their child won't make it through the night. Or about kids who are bullied not for anything they have done to others, but because of their disabilities.

Or a family about to lose their home to foreclosure after losing a job. They don't care about the grass being greener. They're just trying to keep the weeds out.

Too often I have a "sky is falling" approach to life. Glass half empty? Not even! It's broken! And honestly, that is not the person I mean to be. And certainly not the person I want anyone else to think I am. But sometimes when you are in the thick of things, you can't see the light. Fog maybe, but not light. Frustration is a cruel companion. And it's a very close acquaintance of jealously.

Epilogue

CONFUSION HAPPENS

Parenthood isn't a fairytale. Maybe too much Disney and celebrities making big bucks to get photos of their babies on magazine covers have us thinking it will be a piece of cake. Yes, a gazillion dollars, a personal trainer, and a few nannies would get us there. But most of us average, non-famous, underpaid people, are on our own. Kids get sick. Parents scramble for daycare. Spouses fight. Bodies don't go back to the way they were before having children. I'm not saying the sky is falling. But maybe it's a bit cloudy.

But if you've ever felt a lack of purpose in your life, motherhood will fill that gap. You'll have a reason to wake up. Even at 3 am in the morning. You won't be bored. And you'll always have an excuse to go to Target. Ever wonder what to do with all that extra money you earn? No problem. Kids will eat right through that. If you were trying to decide on a career change, parenthood will certainly give you the opportunity to explore your options. You'll be a chef, chauffer, teacher, preacher, personal assistant, maid, seamstress, triage coordinator, entertainer, counselor, and body guard. All at the same time. The pay is close to that of an internship, but hey you'll have purpose.

Motherhood is filled with heartbreak. From watching your baby get shots at doctor visits to seeing them the last ones picked for kickball. They'll stop giving you those daily hugs and tell you they don't need you. They'll challenge your authority and make choices that will have your stomach in knots.

No matter how much you thought you knew before having children, you'll feel less than smart once they're in your life. You will find yourself overwhelmed by the decisions you need to make. Second guessing becomes second nature. *Should I wake her up now, or let her sleep longer? Maybe I should put another blanket over him. Was I supposed to give her a teaspoon or tablespoon of medicine? Is it too soon to look at preschools for him?* It's a never-ending list. It's a list that seems to grow at the same time we are supposed to be sleeping.

Having a child is painful. I mean the actual labor and birth stuff. But veteran mothers will tell you that you forget the pain. It's sort of the same with the not-so-glamorous side of being a mom. Because being a mom will bring you a level of joy that you could have never imagined before. You'll cry happy tears with every milestone. A simple hug will give you more energy than a latte. You'll proudly display art projects even though you don't know what they are. A bad day instantly gets better when your child runs into your arms. Yep. You'll be as sappy as a Sunday afternoon special on the Hallmark channel. Granted that emotion might be cut short when your child tips over the fish bowl, but at least you can take comfort in knowing it was there, which means it can return. And it will. Right after you clean up bits of glass in a pool of water on the floor. And flush the fish down the toilet.

Someone recently told me, “There’s the life that you plan, and then there’s the life that unfolds.” Simple but true. We often try to map out so much of our lives. So then where are we headed as parents? We start at conception and continue on to confusion. Enjoy the ride.

About the Author

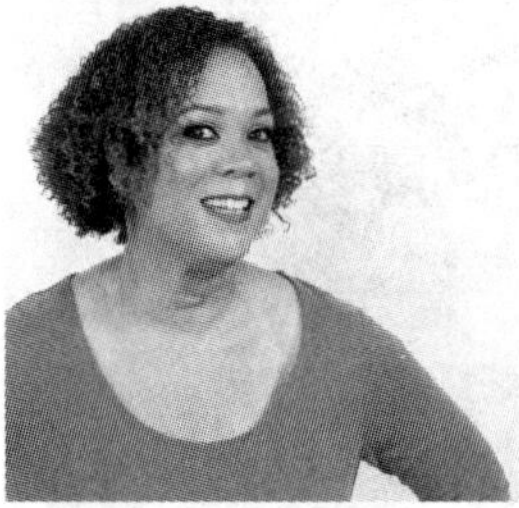

Julie Davidson is an accidental writer from the Midwest. She and her husband, Charles, are raising two teenaged boys. Because she never liked math, she majored in Communication. Julie has spent nearly 20 years as a radio personality where people are forced to listen to her. Additionally, she has written for MetroParent Magazine and the Mommy MD Guide books.

Julie has found through writing and blogging she can connect with others and provide a sense of relief to those who are also confused and frustrated in navigating life's events and relationships. Julie credits her hippy parents and five older brothers for her quirky, sarcastic ways.

When Julie's not writing she dreams of writing from a log cabin in Colorado. And finding out what that foul odor in the house is.

FM funny mommy

- Order our books online
- Purchase them at bookstores nationwide
- Download them for your Kindle, Nook, or iPhone/iPod
- Listen to them on Audible.com

COMING SOON!
WATCH FOR FUTURE TITLES IN THE FUNNY MOMMY SERIES:

12 Months of Gibberish: Surviving Your First Year of Motherhood

Ready, Set, No! Surviving the Toddler Years

Keep It Moving: Losing "Baby Fat" only Applies to Children

Your Life as a Zombie: 100 Reasons to Get Your Baby to Sleep

ALSO BY MOMOSA PUBLISHING LLC

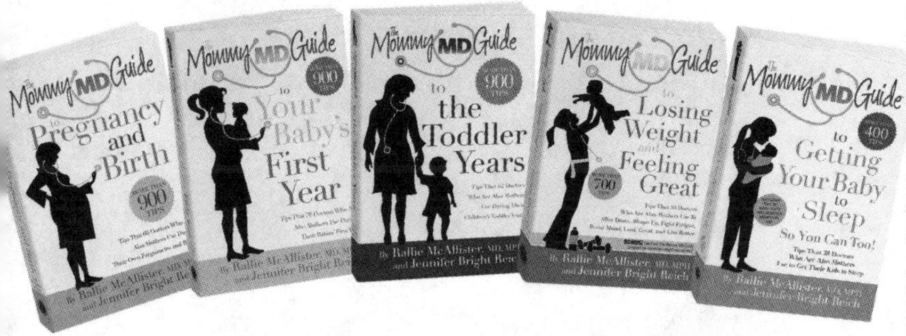

- **Order our books online at many sites, including Walmart.com, Amazon.com, and MommyMDGuides.com**
- **Purchase them at bookstores nationwide**
- **Download them for your Kindle, Nook, or iPhone/iPad**

• • •

Enjoy more Mommy MD Guides' tips on:

The Mommy MD Guide to Pregnancy and Birth app.

Visit us at MommyMDGuides.com
and DaddyMDGuides.com.

COMING SOON!

The Mommy MD Guides are hard at work on more titles in the series. Keep a lookout for:

The Mommy MD Guide to the School Years